The Guide to EKG INTERPRETATION

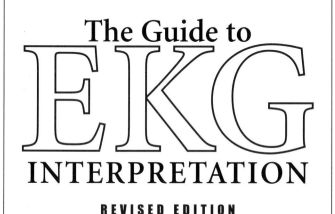

REVISED EDITION

A WHITE COAT POCKET GUIDE

John A. Brose, D.O.
John C. Auseon, D.O.
Daniel Waksman, D.O.
Michael J. Jarosick, D.O.

Ohio University Press
in association with the
Ohio University College of
Osteopathic Medicine

ATHENS

T0132975

Ohio University Press, Athens, Ohio 45701
© 2000 by Ohio University Press
Printed in the United States of America
All rights reserved

20 19 18 17 16 15 14 13 12 11 10   9 8 7 6

Library of Congress Cataloging-in-Publication Data

The guide to EKG interpretation / John A. Brose . . . [et al.].—Rev. ed.
        p. ; cm. — (White coat pocket guide series)
    Includes bibliographical references and index.
    ISBN 0-8214-1328-7 (pbk. : alk. paper)
        1. Electrocardiography—Handbooks, manuals, etc. I. Brose, John A. II. Brose, John A.
    Pocket guide to EKG interpretation. III. Series.
    [DNLM: 1. Electrocardiography—Handbooks. WG 39 G9465 2000]
    RC 683.5.E5 G85 2000
    616.1'207547—dc21

                                                                00-022811

Contents

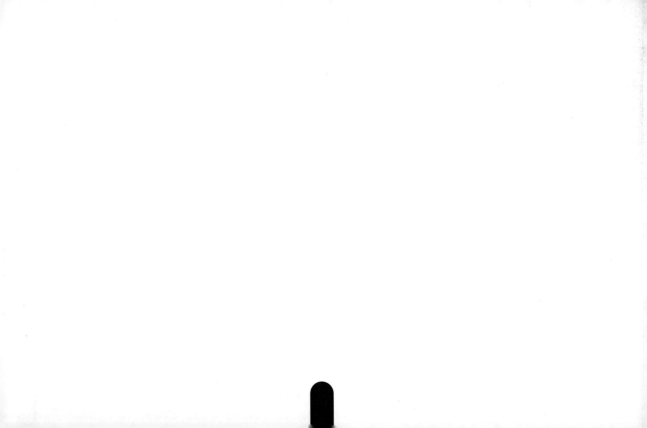

Electrocardiography can be an area of great difficulty for medical students and residents on clinical rotations. Conventional EKG texts are usually too bulky for lab coat pockets. In addition, they often do not approach EKG interpretation in a problem-solving format. While it is easy, therefore, to look up bundle branch block (if one can identify one), placing a diagnosis on a wide QRS complex can be a much more perplexing problem.

This pocket handbook attempts to combine a review of EKG basics with assistance in interpreting EKG abnormalities. In the reading scheme section, students can associate an EKG abnormality (such as QRS widening) with a list of possible diagnoses. Then, using the provided reference page numbers, more complete explanations of these disorders can be obtained.

All EKG examples used in this book were created by translating real or artificially generated EKGs into computer graphic images. The resulting waveforms were then redrawn electronically to accentuate the abnormalities being discussed. The authors wish to express their deep appreciation for the artistic and computer talents of Jeffrey Brown, creator of the illustrations and EKG graphics contained in this book. Our thanks also to Alex Auseon, D.O., and Christine Brose for their assistance in the preparation of the manual.

We hope that you find this handbook useful to you throughout your training.

John A. Brose, D.O.
John C. Auseon, D.O.
Daniel Waksman, D.O.
Michael J. Jarosick, D.O.

Basics of Electrocardiography

Basic Physiology

In order for the myocardium to contract, specialized conduction fibers and the cardiac muscle itself transmit electrical impulses by processes termed "depolarization" and "repolarization." Depolarization implies the electrical activation of a myocardial cell. Repolarization implies a chemical restoration of the cell so that depolarization can be repeated.

The EKG machine utilizes electrodes placed on the arms, legs, and chest which can record this electrical activity of the heart. In some cases there are two electrodes, and the EKG measures the electrical movement between the two. These electrodes are grouped in pairs (one positive and one negative), and are termed "bipolar leads." Included in this category are leads I, II, and III. Other leads utilize a single positive electrode, and measure electrical movement either towards or away from that electrode. These are termed "unipolar leads," and include the limb leads aVR, aVL, aVF, and the precordial leads (V1-V6).

Basic Physiology (cont.)

If a wave of depolarization is approaching a positive electrode, an upward (positive) deflection on the EKG paper is created.

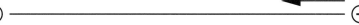

positive complex

If a wave of depolarization is moving away from a positive electrode, a downward (negative) deflection on the EKG paper is created.

negative complex

If a wave of depolarization is moving a right angles to a monitoring electrode, an equiphasic (equally positive and negative) deflection on the EKG is created.

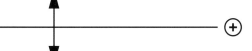

Basics of Electrocardiography

EKG Paper

EKG paper is graph paper divided into small blocks 1 mm square, and larger blocks 5 mm square [each containing twenty-five small blocks (five vertical by five horizontal)]. The height or depth of a deflection is measured in millimeters. Although each small block is one millimeter wide, waves and intervals on an electrocardiogram are measured in seconds rather than in length. Each small block equals 0.04 seconds, and each large block equals 0.2 seconds (five small blocks). Thus, a deflection might be described as 4 mm tall and 0.08 seconds long.

Standard EKG Graph Paper (enlarged for illustration)

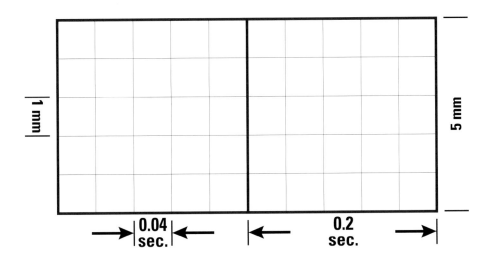

Waves, Complexes, Intervals, and Segments

There are four "waves" that are commonly seen on a normal electrocardiogram. These are termed P wave, T wave, U wave, and QRS complex. Their duration, height, shape, and distances from each other are critical to EKG interpretation. The portion of the EKG tracing between two waves is termed a "segment." If a portion of a tracing includes one or more waves, it is termed an "interval."

Waves:

P wave: This wave represents the electrical activity spreading through the atria.

T wave: Represents part of the recovery (repolarization) phase of the ventricles.

U wave: A small deflection seen after the T wave. Represents the last phase of ventricular repolarization. Large U waves are not normal, and are associated with certain pathological conditions (see p. 51).

Complexes:

QRS Complex: this represents the electrical activity spreading through the ventricles.

Q Wave: If the first portion of the QRS complex is downward in direction, it is a Q wave. If the first portion of the QRS complex is upward in direction, no Q wave is present (no matter how small the upward deflection is).

R Wave: This is the first upward deflection in the QRS complex. If there are two upward deflections, they are termed R and R' (R prime).

S Wave: This is a downward wave that follows an R wave. If there are two downward deflections after an R wave, these are termed S and S' (S prime).

Basics of Electrocardiography

Intervals:

P-R Interval: This interval is measured from the initiation of the P wave to the initiation of the QRS complex. The length of the P-R interval indicates the time taken for an impulse to travel from the atria to the ventricles. The normal P-R interval ranges from 0.12 to 0.20 seconds.

Q-T interval: This interval encompasses the time from the initiation of the QRS complex to the termination of the T wave. It reflects both ventricular depolarization and repolarization. The Q-T interval normally varies with age, sex, and heart rate. The corrected Q-T interval (Q-Tc) can be calculated from the formula:

$$\text{Q-Tc} = \frac{\text{Q-T}}{\sqrt{\text{R-R Interval}}}$$

A normal Q-Tc interval is approximately 0.44±0.02 second

Segments:

P-R segment: This segment encompasses the time from the termination of the P wave to the initiation of the QRS complex. This represents the slowing of conduction across the AV node.

S-T segment: This segment encompasses the distance from the termination of the QRS complex (also known as the J point) to the initiation of the T wave. This represents a portion of the ventricular repolarization. It is important to note that it is the configuration (whether it is elevated or depressed) rather than the absolute measurement of the S-T segment that is used clinically.

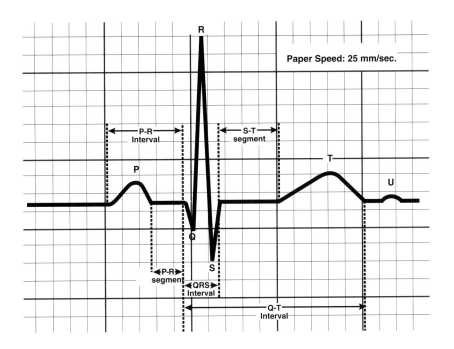

Basics of Electrocardiography

Conduction System of the Heart

The electrical impulses in the normal heart begin in the SA (sinoatrial) node, located in the right atrium. They travel down to the AV (atrioventricular) node via the sinoatrial tracts. This process results in atrial depolarization. The AV node, located on the posterior floor of the right atrium, then slows the impulse to allow ventricular filling. After traversing the AV node, the impulse spreads rapidly down the bundle of His and through the right and left bundle branches, depolarizing the septum and the ventricles.

There are two main bundle branches, termed the "right" and the "left." The right bundle branch supplies the right ventricle. The left bundle branch has two divisions, termed the "anterior" and "posterior" fascicles. The anterior fascicle spreads superiorly in the left ventricle, while the posterior fascicle spreads inferiorly. Abnormalities in this system are discussed in the section on "bundle branch block" (p. 70) and "fascicular block" (p. 78).

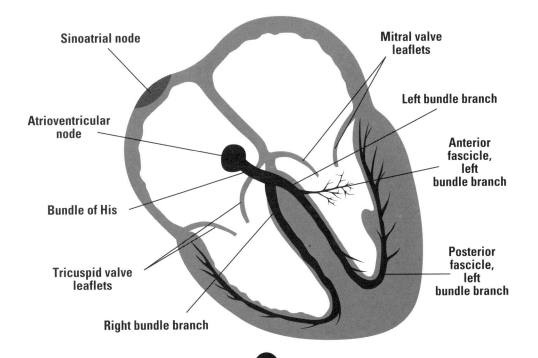

Sinoatrial node

Mitral valve
leaflets

Left bundle branch

Atrioventricular
node

Anterior
fascicle,
left
bundle branch

Bundle of His

Posterior
fascicle,
left
bundle branch

Tricuspid valve
leaflets

Right bundle branch

Basics of Electrocardiography

12 Standard EKG Leads

Limb Leads: these leads examine the electrical activity of the heart in a "frontal plane," giving information about electrical movement superiorly, inferiorly, right and left.

Leads I, II, and III: these leads are bipolar (include both a positive and negative electrode), with electrodes placed on the arms and legs. Although multiple electrodes are attached to the patient simultaneously, the EKG machine uses only two electrodes at a time.

Lead I: a negative electrode is placed on the right arm, a positive electrode on the left arm.

Lead II: a negative electrode is placed on the right arm, a positive electrode on the left foot.

Lead III: a negative electrode is placed on the left arm, a positive electrode on the left foot.

Electrocardiographic Leads - Limb Leads

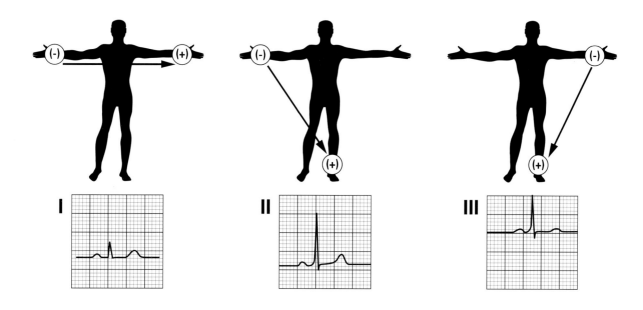

Leads aVR, aVL, and aVF: these unipolar leads (single positive electrode) are termed "augmented," because the amplitude of the deflections is electrically increased by changing the connections within the EKG machine. The electrode is always positive, and is named after its location (thus, aVF refers to an Augmented Voltage lead with the positive electrode on the Foot. The "negative" pole is interpreted by the machine as being between the right arm and the left arm).

Lead aVR: a positive electrode is placed on the right arm. The negative pole bisects the left arm and the left foot.

Lead aVL: a positive electrode is placed on the left arm. The negative pole bisects the right arm and the left foot.

Lead aVF: a positive electrode is placed on the left foot. The negative pole bisects the right arm and the left arm.

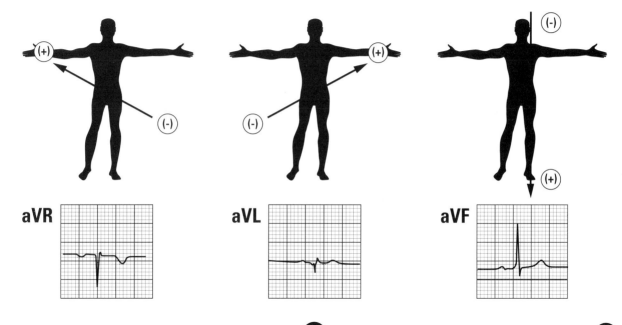

aVR aVL aVF

Basics of Electrocardiography

Precordial (Chest) Leads:

These unipolar leads are placed on specific areas across the chest as specified in the diagram on the next page. They examine the electrical activity of the heart in a horizontal plane, giving information about electrical movement anteriorly, posteriorly, right and left. Abnormal progression of the QRS complex across the precordium can be of great clinical importance. Normal R wave progression begins with a small R wave and a large S wave in V1; as one progresses along the precordial leads, the R wave should become progressively larger while the S wave becomes smaller as you approach lead V5 or V6. The S wave may indeed be nonexistent in V6. The normal area of transition where the R wave becomes larger than the S wave is in either leads V3 or V4.

There are certain situations when it is helpful to use additional leads other than the standard leads. Examples of these are the X, Y, and Z leads, also known as orthogonal leads.

Lead X: a positive electrode is placed in the left axilla and a negative electrode is placed in the right axilla. This lead will therefore demonstrate forces that are going either right-to-left or left-to-right.

Lead Y: a positive electrode is placed on the front of the lower part of the chest and a negative electrode is placed on the neck. This lead will therefore demonstrate forces that proceed in an up-down direction.

Lead Z: a positive electrode is placed on the anterior part of the chest and a negative electrode is placed on the back. This lead will therefore demonstrate the approximate equivalent of an inverted lead V2.

Precordial (Anterior) Leads

The six precordial leads are unipolar leads and view the electrical activity of the heart in the horizontal plane.

The leads are placed as follows:

- **V1** 4th intercostal space immediately to the right of the sternum
- **V2** 4th intercostal space immediately to the left of the sternum
- **V3** Directly between V2 and V4
- **V4** 5th intercostal space — left midclavicular line
- **V5** 5th intercostal space — left anterior axillary line
- **V6** 5th intercostal space — left midaxillary line

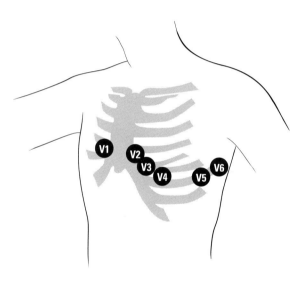

Precordial Leads (cont.)

It is sometimes helpful to place precordial leads on the right side of the chest. These leads are named V1R, V2R, V3R, etc. These leads measure right-sided electrical activity in a horizontal plane.

Einthoven's Triangle and the Hexaxial System

The three limb leads can be placed together to form "Einthoven's Triangle" as shown. If these leads are then rearranged so that they converge in a common point, the hexaxial diagram is created (see p. 21). The "arms" of the hexaxial diagram have arbitrarily been assigned degrees. The general direction of electrical current flow in the heart, or axis, can be plotted on this chart. The method of computing axis is discussed beginning on p. 20.

EINTHOVEN'S TRIANGLE

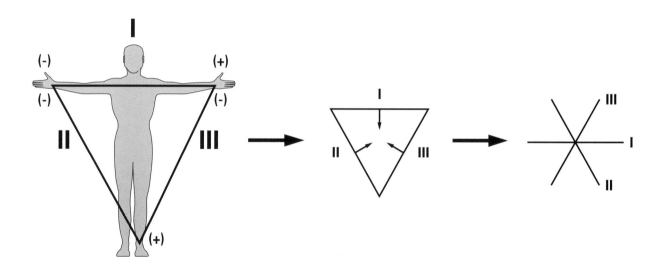

19

I

Axis Determination

Axis Determination

Axis is most simply viewed as the general direction of the heart's electrical activity. Although P waves and T waves have their own axis, determining axis usually refers to only the QRS axis. Calculation of the QRS axis is helpful in diagnosing a variety of conditions, including ventricular hypertrophy (see p. 62) and hemiblocks (see p. 78).

For general purposes, it may be stated that a normal axis lies between 0 and 90 degrees. However, there is some disagreement concerning what constitutes a normal axis. Most authors would agree that an axis beyond -30 degrees to the left or beyond +105 degrees to the right would be abnormal. An axis between 0 and -30 degrees might be termed "slight left axis deviation."

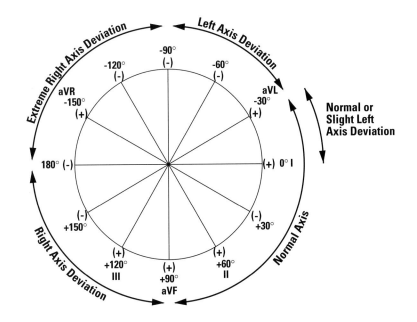

Axis Determination

Computation of Axis; Approximate and Exact Methods

Calculation of Approximate Axis: In order to determine approximate axis, a three-step process is recommended. In the vast majority of clinical situations, an approximate axis is all that is needed. It is emphasized that computation of axis is based only upon the limb leads (I, II, III, aVR, aVL, aVF). The precordial leads (VI-V6) are not used in axis determination.

Step 1: Examine leads I and aVF. Determine whether the QRS complex is primarily positive (total upward deflection exceeds total downward deflection) or negative (total downward deflection exceeds total upward deflection) in these two leads.

-If I and aVF are both positive, the axis is normal (between 0 and +90 degrees).
-If I is positive and aVF is negative, there is <u>left</u> axis deviation (between 0 and -90 degrees).
-If I is negative and aVF is positive, there is <u>right</u> axis deviation (between +90 and +180 degrees).
-If both I and aVF are negative, the axis is in "no man's land" (between +180 and -90 degrees).

Note: Many clinicians prefer to use lead II rather than lead aVF as a rapid reference lead. Hence, if leads I and II are both positive, the axis lies between -30° and +90°. If lead I is positive and lead II is negative, there is left axis deviation between -30° and -90°. This method is particularly useful for rapid determination if one considers the normal range to be +90° to -30°.

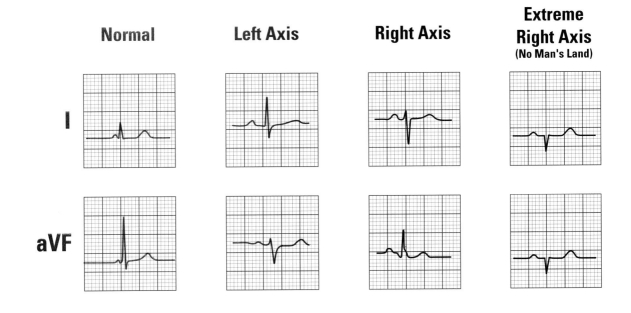

Axis Determination

Step 2: Now that the correct quadrant has been determined, computing the axis in approximate degrees is required.

-Find the limb lead that is most nearly equiphasic (the QRS is equally positive and negative). The axis lies at right angles to this lead. Refer back to step one to determine which quadrant the axis lies in.

Note: The equiphasic lead usually has the smallest total deflection of any of the limb leads. Conversely, if the axis lies directly along a lead, that lead will generally have the largest deflection of any of the limb leads (either positive or negative, depending on the axis).

-If there are two leads that appear to be almost equiphasic, the axis generally lies at right angles to the point between these two leads.

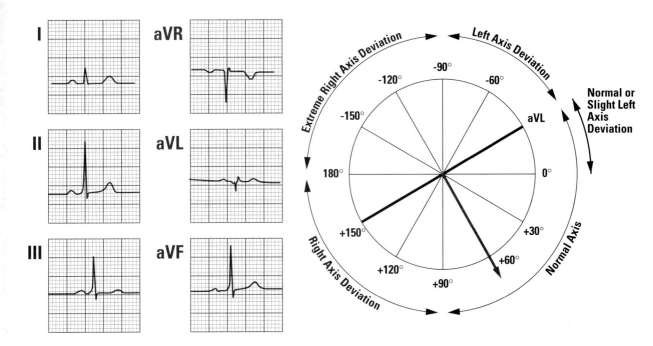

Step 3: Having arrived at an approximate axis, fine adjustment is sometimes required. If there is a lead that is exactly equiphasic, then the axis lies at right angles to this lead and no further refinement is necessary. If the chosen equiphasic lead is not *exactly* equiphasic, however, a closer estimation can be made as follows:

-If the equiphasic lead is a little more positive than negative, move the axis proportionally towards the *positive* pole of the equiphasic lead. If the equiphasic lead is a little more negative than positive, move the axis proportionally towards the *negative* pole of the equiphasic lead.

Note: Occasionally there may be EKGs where all of the limb leads appear to be equiphasic. Since a correct axis cannot be determined, this is termed an "indeterminate" axis.

Example: More Precise Axis Determination

Lead aVL

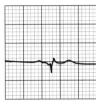

The nearly equiphasic lead is more negative than positive, therefore, shift the axis towards negative aVL, but do not exceed 75°. (If the axis exceeded 75°, a different lead should be equiphasic.)

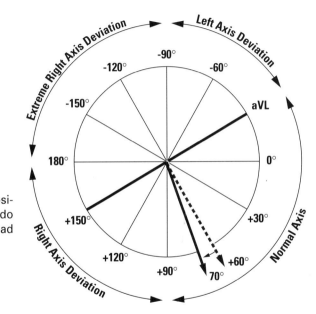

Axis Determination

Exact Determination of Axis: As noted previously, it is seldom necessary to determine the exact axis. If it is desired to do so, however, the method is as follows:

-Look at lead I. Compute the area under the positive deflection of the QRS complex by using the formula (area = 1/2 base x height). Do the same for the negative deflection, and add the positive and the negative areas together. Plot the value obtained on the hexaxial diagram along lead I.

Note: Normally, the width of the QRS will be the same in leads I and III. Therefore, the heights of the QRS complexes can be substituted for the areas when plotting the points along the leads, making computation easier. Don't forget to add the negative deflection (a negative number) to the positive deflection to obtain the total deflection.

Step 1: Exact Axis Determination

Lead I

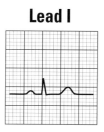

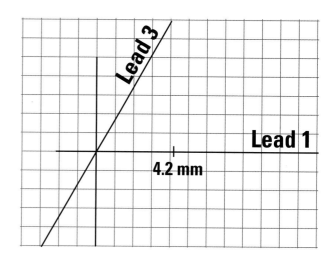

4.2 mm

-Next, look at lead III. Compute the area under the positive deflection of the QRS complex by using the formula (area = 1/2 base x height). Do the same for the negative deflection, and add the positive and the negative areas together. Plot the value obtained on the hexaxial diagram along lead III.

Note: Normally, the width of the QRS will be the same in leads I and III. Therefore, the heights of the QRS complexes can be substituted for the areas when plotting the points along the leads, making computation easier. Don't forget to add the negative deflection (a negative number) to the positive deflection to obtain the total deflection.

-Draw lines through the plotted points at right angles to the respective leads. The point at which these lines intersect is the exact axis.

Step 2: Exact Axis Determination

Lead I

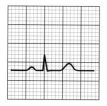

Deflection (+)4.2 mm

Plot point on Lead I

Lead III

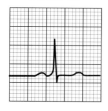

Upward deflection	+10.0
Downward deflection	-1.6
Net deflection	+8.4

Plot point on Lead III

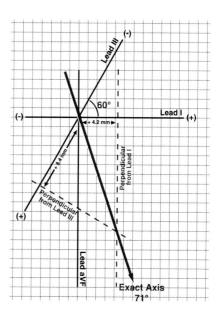

Heart Rate Determination

The heart rate can be determined from the EKG tracing using several different methods. Each of these methods has advantages in certain clinical situations. The paper speed must be set at 25 mm/sec. for these methods to be accurate. Today, most EKG machines compute the heart rate automatically.

Determination of the rate by counting large blocks

The rate can be easily calculated by counting the number of large blocks between two QRS complexes, and dividing that number into 300. Thus, if there are six large blocks between two QRS complexes, the rate is 50 beats per minute. If the QRS spikes do not fall exactly on the edge of a large box, an exact rate can be obtained by adding the number of large boxes plus the number of small boxes (each counting as 0.2 of a large box), and dividing the sum into 300. Therefore if the distance between two QRS spikes is five large boxes and four small boxes, the calculation would be 300 divided by 5.8, or 52 beats per minute. This is a very accurate method, but is time consuming.

Determination of the rate by large blocks and number pattern

To determine the rate more rapidly, it is useful to memorize the number pattern "300, 150, 100, 75, 60, 50, 43." Each of these numbers is then applied to a large box between two QRS complexes. Thus, if there are four large boxes between QRS spikes, one would count "300, 150, 100, 75," giving a rate of 75 beats per minute. If the rate falls below 50, another method must be used. If a spike falls between lines, an approximation must be made (e.g., if spike falls between 100 and 150, the approximate rate would be 125).

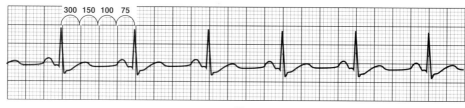

Heart rate: 75 beats per minute

Heart Rate Determination

Determination of the rate by three-second marks

Sometimes in emergency situations, a very rapid method of determining rate is necessary. If there is profound bradycardia, using the previous two methods can be difficult. At the top of EKG paper there are small vertical marks at three-second intervals. A quick approximation of rate can be obtained by counting the number of cardiac cycles in a six-second interval and multiplying by ten. Thus, if there are three complete cardiac cycles between the first and the third three-second marks, the heart rate is 30 beats per minute.

EKG rulers

Many inexpensive EKG rulers are available that assist in computing rate. One simply places the ruler on the electrocardiogram noting where the designated QRS spikes fall on the ruler. Usually, two QRS cycles are measured, and the rate is then read directly off the ruler (see following page).

Use of Heart Rate Ruler

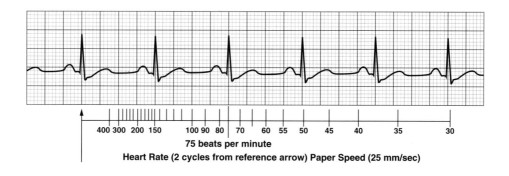

75 beats per minute

Heart Rate (2 cycles from reference arrow) Paper Speed (25 mm/sec)

To ensure a thorough EKG analysis, it is necessary to employ a systematic reading scheme. The reader is encouraged to choose from several published schemes or to develop his/her own. The scheme that has proven effective for these authors is one that begins with the *P wave* and moves to the right examining the segments, intervals, and wave forms as they occur chronologically. First, rate (p. 32) and rhythm are determined and then the above-mentioned analysis is performed for the identification of other abnormalities.

Specifically, the components examined in order are the *P wave, P-R interval, QRS complex, QRS axis, S-T segment, T wave, U wave, and Q-T interval.* These components need to be examined in all leads. A detailed description of how to perform this analysis follows. When an abnormality is encountered, the reader is given a list of differentials to consider as an explanation for the abnormal finding. Practice will make this process automatic.

1. P Wave

The normal P wave should be:
> *-of uniform appearance within each lead.*
> *-no taller than 2.5 mm.*
> *-no wider than 0.12 seconds (3 small blocks).*
> *-positive (upward deflection) in lead II.*
> *-negative (downward deflection) in lead aVR.*

Common variations of P waves:
*Examine the P wave for uniformity and regularity.
> -Consider: PACs (Premature Atrial Contractions) (p. 154).
> Wandering pacemaker (p. 166).
> Multifocal atrial tachycardia.

*Examine whether there is a relation of the P wave to the QRS complex.

*Examine the P waves for deformity.

Reading Scheme

*Examine size and shape of P wave.
-Is it tall (> 2.5 mm vertical displacement) and/or narrow?
-Consider: Right atrial enlargement (p. 56).
May be due to conduction abnormality.
-Is it wide (> 0.12 sec.) and /or biphasic?
-Consider: Atrial enlargement (p. 56).
Accelerated paper speed (50 mm/sec.).
-Is it wide and/or notched?
-Consider: Left atrial enlargement (p. 58).
May be due to conduction abnormality.

*Examine for inversion in leads II and aVR.
-Inversion in these leads (negative in II and positive in aVR) can be indicative of retrograde depolarization of the atria which occurs in some cases of junctional rhythm (p. 168). If this occurs, the P-R interval will be short (< 0.12 sec). Recall that in junctional rhythm P waves are absent in most leads and may be absent in all leads (p. 168).

*Evaluate proximity of the P wave to the QRS complex. This is done by measuring the P-R interval which is defined as the length of time from the beginning of the P wave to the beginning of the QRS complex (see p. 9).

-Is P wave present or absent? If absent:
   -Consider: Premature ventricular contraction (p. 182).
                Atrial flutter (p. 162).
                Atrial fibrillation (p. 162).
                Junctional rhythm (p. 172).
                Ventricular rhythm (p. 188).
                Sinoatrial arrest.
-Is there more than one P wave per QRS complex?
   -Consider: Heart block:
                Atrial Tachycardia with block (p. 158).
                Second degree AV block (p. 210).
                Third degree AV block (p. 214).
                Atrial flutter (p. 162).
                Atrial fibrillation (p. 164).

Reading Scheme

2. P-R Interval

The normal P-R interval should be:
-between 0.12 and 0.20 seconds in duration.
-choose the longest P-R interval in a limb lead for measurement.

*Examine the length of the P-R interval.
   -Is it <u>prolonged</u> (longer than 0.20 seconds)?
      -Consider: Atrioventricular block (p. 208).
                  Chronic aortic regurgitation.
                  Drug effects [Digitalis toxicity (p. 92)].
                  AV block.

   -Is it <u>shortened</u> (shorter than 0.12 seconds)?
      -Consider: Junctional rhythm (p. 168).
                  Tachycardia.
                  Pre-excitation syndromes:
                     Wolff-Parkinson-White syndrome (p. 112).
                     Lown-Ganong-Levine syndrome (p. 114).
                  Normal variant in a child.
                  Normal variant in an adult.

3. QRS Complex

If review is necessary see QRS nomenclature (p. 7) and definition of Q, R, and S waves (p. 7).

The normal QRS complex should be:
  -of uniform appearance within each lead.
  -no wider than 0.12 sec. (it is usually < 0.10 sec.).
  -free of significant Q waves (p. 43).
  -distinctly separate from the P wave.
  The remaining "normal" characteristics of the QRS complex vary with lead placement.
Other characteristics of QRS complexes will be discussed on the following page.

*Examine QRS for uniformity of appearance within each lead.
  -Is there variation (some complexes appearing wide and bizarre)?
    -Consider ventricular ectopy:
                PVCs (p. 180).
                Ventricular escape beats (p. 195).
                Idioventricular rhythm in AV dissociation (p. 202).
                Ventricular tachycardia.
                Accelerated ventricular tachycardia.

*Examine width of QRS in the limb leads.
  -Is QRS uniform within each lead but abnormally wide (>0.12 sec.)?
    -Consider: Bundle Branch Block (p. 72).
                Intraventricular conduction defect (p. 74).
                Electronic paced rhythm (gives bundle branch block appearance) (p. 74).
                Wolff-Parkinson-White syndrome (p. 112).
                Drug effects (p. 86).
                Hyperkalemia (p. 96).
                Idioventricular rhythm (p. 196).
                Increased paper speed on EKG machine.
                Aberrant ventricular conduction.
                Fusion beats.

*Examine all leads (except aVR) for significant Q waves.

A significant Q wave is:

    1) >1 mm wide, i.e. >1 small square, i.e. >0.04 sec. duration

                    -or-

    2) > or = 1/3 (some authors say 1/4) of the total vertical magnitude of the QRS.

    3) A QS complex is always significant except in lead aVR.

Note: *Small Q waves are commonly present in I, II, V5, V6 and are considered non-pathologic. Q waves are commonly absent in most leads.*

-Are there any significant Q waves?

    -Consider: Infarction (p. 120).

                 Wolf-Parkinson-White syndrome (p. 112).

                 Bundle branch block.

-Note the leads which have the significant Q waves to localize the infarction (p. 120).

-Although the significant Q wave is the hallmark of acute transmural MI, it is also necessary to examine the S-T segment and the T wave in order to completely evaluate ischemia (p. 120), injury (p. 122), and infarction (p. 124).

Reading Scheme

4. S-T Segment

Represents the beginning of ventricular repolarization. Begins at the termination of the QRS complex and ends at the beginning of the T wave (see p. 9). The J-point is defined as the point at which the S-T segment "takes off" from the QRS complex.

The normal S-T Segment should be:
> *-isoelectric, i.e., on the baseline (should not deviate by more than 1 mm from the baseline).*

*Examine the position of the S-T Segment.
  -Is the S-T segment <u>depressed</u>?
    -Consider: Subendocardial ischemia/injury (p. 128).
                Non-Q wave infarction (p. 128).
                Hypertrophy and/or "strain" pattern (p. 62).
                Reciprocal changes with Q wave MI (p. 142).
                Digitalis effect (p. 90).
                Quinidine effect (p. 86).
                Hypokalemia (p. 94).

-Is the S-T segment <u>elevated</u>?

-Consider: Injury pattern (p. 122).

Q wave (transmural) MI - acute (see pages 121-140).

Early repolarization variant - this may be normal for healthy, young adult patients, particularly in black patients (see pp. 115-116).

Prinzmetal's angina.

Ventricular aneurysm (see pp. 103-104).

Acute pericarditis (p. 102).

Epicardial injury.

Post-myocardial infarction syndrome (Dressler's syndrome). This may be chronic in VI and V2 when associated with LVH and LBBB (see pp. 73-74).

Hypothermia (p. 102).

Reading Scheme

Tips in evaluating S-T segment abnormalities:

*Examine all leads when evaluating the S-T segment. This is helpful in differential diagnosis.

In <u>early repolarization</u> the S-T segment elevation is usually prominent in the chest leads (V4-V6). This elevation is stable over time; i.e., you do **not** see the evolving sequence of ST-T changes seen with acute pericarditis and MI.

In <u>acute pericarditis</u> the S-T segment elevation is more diffuse; i.e., it is more likely seen in all leads (remember: the pericardium surrounds the heart). This elevation is followed by T wave inversion as the S-T segment returns to the baseline. In comparison to MI, there are **no** abnormal Q waves and **no** reciprocal changes.

In <u>MI</u> the S-T segment elevation is more localized, reflecting the exact area of heart muscle that infarcted. This elevation is also followed by T wave inversion as the S-T segment returns to the baseline. With a transmural MI, one **finds** abnormal Q waves and often the presence of reciprocal changes (p. 142).

5. T Wave

Represents part of ventricular repolarization (see p. 9).

The normal T wave should be:
> *-of the same direction as the main deflection of the QRS complexes in all leads.*
> *-positive (upward deflection) in leads II, V3-V6.*
> *-negative (downward deflection) in lead aVR.*
> *-variable in all other leads; III, aVL, aVF, V1.*
> *-asymmetric; the peak is closer to the end of the wave than to the beginning.*
> *-not >5 mm in limb leads and not >10 mm in precordial leads.*

*Examine the direction of the T wave.
  -Is it abnormally inverted?
     -Consider: Myocardial ischemia (p. 120).

                    Q wave MI — evolving (p. 124).
                    Non-Q wave infarction (p. 128).
                    May be normal in children.
                    Ventricular aneurysm (p. 106).
                    Acute pericarditis (p. 102).
                    Pulmonary embolus (p. 108).
                    Digitalis effect (p. 90).
                    Persistent "juvenile T wave inversion" pattern; mostly in females; seen in right chest leads, V1-V3.
                    CVA - particularly subarachnoid hemorrhage (p. 116).
                    Hypertrophy and/or "strain" pattern (p. 62).
                    Post-tachycardia T wave syndrome.
                    Post-pacemaker T wave pattern.
                    Early repolarization variant (p. 118).
                    Severe myxedema.
                    RBBB/LBBB (p. 72).
                    Mitral valve prolapse.
                    Acute abdominal problems (especially acute pancreatitis).

*Examine the shape of the T wave.
  -Is it notched?
      -Consider: This may be normal in children.
                 Quinidine effect (p. 86).
                 Acute pericarditis (p. 102).
  -Is it symmetrical?
      -Consider: MI (p. 124).
                 Hyperkalemia (p. 96).
                 Myocarditis.

*Examine the height of the T wave.
  -Is it tall and peaked?
      -Consider: Acute Q wave MI (p. 124).
                 Hyperkalemia (p. 96).
                 Myocardial ischemia (p. 120).
                 CVA (p. 116).
                 Diastolic overloading, such as pure aortic insufficiency, mitral insufficiency, and left to right
                    shunts.

-Is the T wave flat or depressed?

    -Consider: Hypokalemia (p. 94).

                Hypertrophy and/or "strain" pattern (p. 62).

                Myocarditis.

                Type I antiarrhythmics, e.g., Quinidine, Procainamide, Disopyramide.

                Digitalis effect (p. 90).

                Myxedema.

                Chronic pericarditis (p. 102).

                Pericardial effusion.

                Hypopituitarism.

                Phenothiazines.

                Tricyclic antidepressants.

6. U Wave

This wave is not always seen; when it is seen, it is usually small and of low voltage. If present, it is found after the T wave. Represents the last phase of ventricular repolarization. Coincides with the phase of supernormal excitability during ventricular recovery, thus this is when most premature ventricular beats occur. Is best discerned in lead V3.

The normal U wave should be:
> *-in the same direction as the T wave.*

*Examine its direction.
  -Is it in the opposite direction of the T wave?
    -Consider: LVH and/or "strain" pattern (p. 64).
              Myocardial ischemia (coronary insufficiency) (p. 120).

*Examine its shape.
  -Is the U wave prominent?
      -Consider: Hypokalemia (p. 94).
                    Quinidine effect (p. 86).
                    Digitalis effect (p. 90).
                    Hypercalcemia (p. 100).
                    Thyrotoxicosis.
                    Epinephrine.
                    CVA (will be inverted if T wave is also inverted) (p. 116).
                    Phenothiazines.
                    Tricyclic antidepressants.
                    Procainamide.
                    Disopyramide effect.
                    Exercise.

7. Q-T Interval

The normal Q-T interval should be:
> *-Corrected for heart rate using either Q-Tc calculation or a corrected Q-T table. The Q-Tc can vary according to age and sex. A rule of thumb: Q-T interval should not be more than one-half the length of the R-R interval when a sinus rhythm is present. This pertains only to rates between 65-90 beats per minute.*

*Examine length of the Q-T interval.
  -Is it prolonged?
      -Consider: Congenital Q-T prolongation.
                  Hypocalcemia (p. 98).
                  Type I antiarrhythmics (i.e., quinidine, procainamide).
                  Hyperkalemia (p. 96).
                  Rheumatic fever.
                  Congestive heart failure.
                  Mitral valve prolapse.
                  Hypothermia (p. 104).
                  Myocarditis.
                  Artifact (EKG paper running at double speed).

  -Is it shortened?
      -Consider: Digitalis effect (p. 90).
                  Hypercalcemia (p. 100).
                  Hyperkalemia (p. 96).

Chamber Hypertrophy/Enlargement

Hypertrophy

Enlargement of a chamber of the heart may be the result of dilatation of the chamber or it may be due to an increase in the chamber wall thickness. The latter represents correct usage of the term hypertrophy. However, the term is often used interchangeably with enlargement of a chamber by either of the two mechanisms. The characteristic EKG changes that occur for a given chamber enlargement will be the same regardless of which type of enlargement is present. A description of the characteristic EKG findings for enlargement of each of the four chambers follows.

V

Right Atrial Enlargement (RAE)

The P wave configuration in RAE is often referred to as **P-pulmonale** because it is characteristic of chronic cor pulmonale. Cor pulmonale is a disease characterized by pathologic changes in the heart (enlargement of right atrium and ventricle) due to pressure overload. This is caused by increased pulmonary circuit resistance associated with severe pulmonary disease. A transient p-pulmonale pattern may reflect an acute process such as an asthma attack or pulmonary embolism (situations in which sudden increases in pulmonary resistance can occur). The term **P-congenitale** is used when RAE is the result of congenital heart disease.

EKG Findings

-Tall, narrow P waves (≥2.5 mm height) in leads II, III, aVF. Lead II is most sensitive for this finding.
-Width of P wave is not increased.
-Less commonly, there is a ≥2 mm upright component of P wave in V1 or V2.

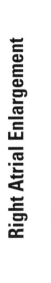

Right Atrial Enlargement

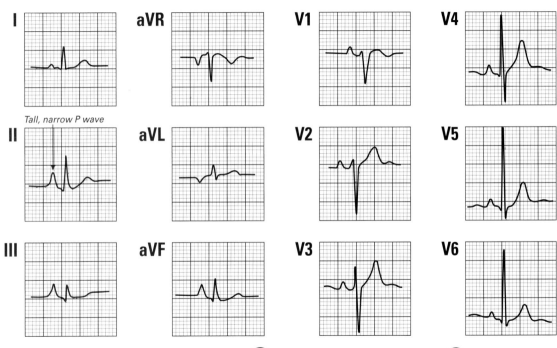

I

II

Tall, narrow P wave

III

aVR

aVL

aVF

V1

V2

V3

V4

V5

V6

V

Left Atrial Enlargement (LAE)

The P wave configuration of LAE is often called **P-mitrale** because it is associated with mitral valve disease.

EKG Findings

-P waves are wide (≥3 mm [0.12 sec.]) and notched in one or more limb leads (especially I, II, aVL).

-P waves of V1 and V2 may have negative terminal component with depth and width ≥1 mm.

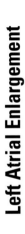

Left Atrial Enlargement

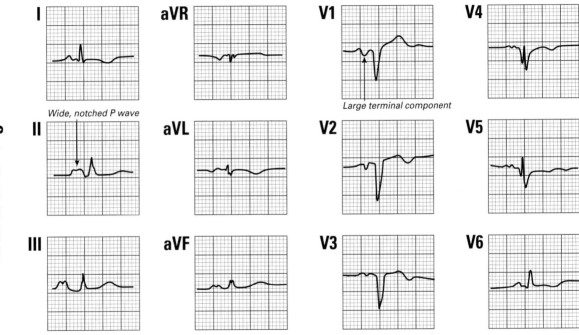

I

aVR

V1

V4

Wide, notched P wave

II

aVL

V2

V5

Large terminal component

III

aVF

V3

V6

59

V

Biatrial Enlargement

EKG Findings
-Findings for both RAE and LAE.

RAE
-Tall, narrow P waves (≥ 2.5 mm height) in leads II, III, aVF. Lead II is most sensitive for this finding.
-Width of P wave is not increased.
-Less commonly, there is a ≥2 mm upright component of the P wave in V1 or V2.

LAE
-P waves are wide (≥3 mm [0.12 sec.]) and notched in one or more limb leads (especially I, II, aVL).
-P waves of V1 and V2 may have negative terminal component with depth and width ≥1 mm.

Biatrial Enlargement

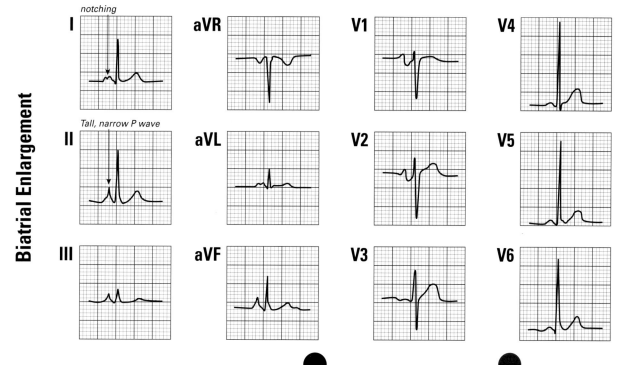

V

Right Ventricular Hypertrophy (RVH)

Because the mass (and hence the magnitude of depolarization) of the LV greatly exceeds that of the RV in the normal heart, RVH must be profound in order for EKG changes to be apparent. These EKG changes can be conceptualized as a reversal in the usual pattern of LV over RV dominance. Initially, there is a progressive axis deviation to the right. This change is followed by reduction of S wave magnitude in V1 with a resultant increase in the R:S ratio in that lead.

EKG Findings

-RAD $\geq 90°$ (unless concurrent LVH is also present).
-R wave > S wave magnitude in V1 (R:S>1 in V1).
—or—
R wave magnitude in V1 + S wave magnitude in V6 $\geq$ 11mm.
-Deep S waves may be present in V5-V6, I, aVL.
-RR' pattern may be present in V1.
-Often present are secondary repolarization changes known as "RV Strain Pattern," i.e., S-T depression and asymmetric T wave inversion in right chest leads and some limb leads. The depressed S-T segment will have an upward convexity in leads with positive QRS complexes.

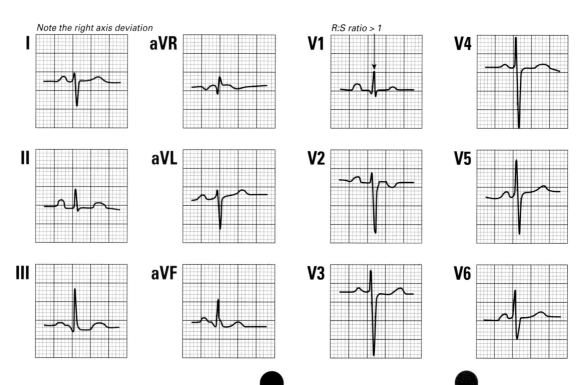

Note the right axis deviation

R:S ratio > 1

I aVR V1 V4

II aVL V2 V5

III aVF V3 V6

63

V

Left Ventricular Hypertrophy (LVH)

Because the mass (and hence magnitude of depolarization) of the LV greatly exceeds that of the RV in the normal heart, some of the EKG changes in LVH are simply exaggerations of the normal pattern of LV dominance. For example, tall R waves in left precordial leads become taller and deep S waves in right precordial leads become deeper. It is useful to envision this trend before attempting to memorize specific criteria.

Left Ventricular Hypertrophy (cont.)

EKG Findings which may be seen with LVH

-S wave in V1 + R wave in V5 or V6 ≥ 35 mm.

-R wave in V5 or V6 ≥ 26 mm.

-R wave in aVL ≥ 13 mm.

-Often present are secondary repolarization changes known as "LV Strain Pattern," i.e., S-T depression and asymmetric T wave inversion in the left chest leads and limb leads that have tall R waves. The depressed S-T segment will have an upward convexity in leads with positive QRS complexes. The classic "LV Strain Pattern" occurs in LVH secondary to systolic overload. If the LVH is instead associated with diastolic overload, T waves will be tall, narrow, and upright rather than inverted.

-Sometimes widening of the QRS complex may be seen (it takes more time for depolarization to spread through a thickened myocardium). The delayed onset of intrinsicoid deflection (≥0.045 sec) is responsible for the increased QRS duration. Intrinsicoid deflection refers to the measurement from the onset of the QRS complex to the peak of the R wave.

-LAD may be present.

Note: EKG representation of LVH is quite variable and, as a result, several sets of criteria and scoring systems have been developed in an attempt to increase the sensitivity of this difficult EKG diagnosis. On the following page are listed the popular **Estes-Romhilt Point Score System** and the **Cornell Voltage Criteria**.

Left Ventricular Hypertrophy (cont.)

Cornell Voltage Criteria for EKG Diagnosis of LVH
   -Men: S in V3 + R in aVL > 28 mm.   **-Women:** S in V3 + R in aVL > 20 mm.
(Ref. Casale, P.N., Devereux R.B., Alonso D.R., Campo E., Kligfield P.: Improved sex-specific criteria of left ventricular hypertrophy for clinical and computer interpretation of electrocardiograms: validation with autopsy findings. Circulation, 1987; 75(3): 565-572).

Estes-Romhilt Point Score System
1. R or S in limb lead:	20 mm or more	
S in V1, V2, or V3	25 mm or more	3 pts.
R in V4, V5, or V6	25 mm or more	
2. Any ST shift (without digitalis)		3 pts.
Typical "strain" ST-T (with digitalis)		1 pt.
3. LAD: -15° or more		2 pts.
4. QRS interval: 0.09 sec. or more		1 pt.
5. Intrinsicoid Deflection in V5-6: 0.04 sec. or more		1 pt.
6. P-terminal force in V1 more than 0.04		3 pts.
TOTAL		**13 pts.**

   (5=LVH; 4=probable LVH)
(Ref. Romhilt, D.W., and Estes, E.H.: A point-score system for ECG diagnosis of left ventricular hypertrophy. Am. Heart J., 6: 752, 1968).

Left Ventricular Hypertrophy (LVH)

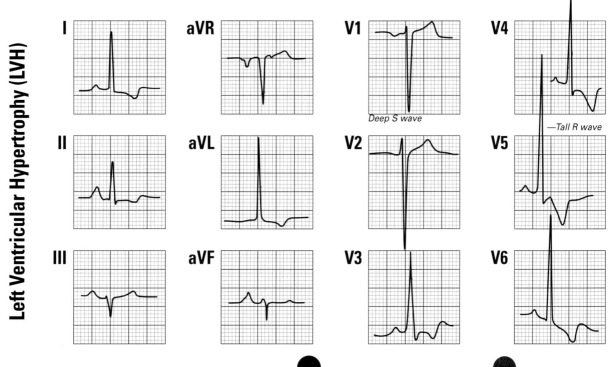

Biventricular Hypertrophy

Recognizing biventricular hypertrophy by EKG is difficult due to the tendency of RVH and LVH EKG changes to neutralize each other. Furthermore, presentation is quite variable. Descriptions of the most likely patterns follow.

EKG Findings

-LVH per chest leads (voltage criteria) + RAD per limb leads; **AND/OR**:

-LVH per chest leads (voltage criteria) + prominent R waves in right chest leads; **AND/OR**:

-shallow S wave in V1 + strikingly deeper S in V2; **AND/OR**:

-relatively equiphasic RS pattern in midleft chest leads; **AND/OR**:

-RVH per chest leads (voltage criteria) + LAD per limb leads; **AND/OR**:

-relatively tall R waves in all chest leads.

On EKG below, note:

Right axis deviation (p. 20).

Tall, peaked P waves suggestive of right atrial enlargement (p. 65).

LVH by voltage criteria (p. 65).

Biventricular Hypertrophy

Note: See previous page

I   aVR   V1   V4

II   aVL   V2   V5

III   aVF   V3   V6

Blocks

Delays (also known as "blocks") can occur in the special conduction system within the heart. When these abnormalities are present, there are resultant changes in the direction and timing of depolarization. The EKG manifestations of these changes are specific to the location of the block.

Blocks in the AV node and bundle of His (AV bundle) result in rhythm disturbances or prolongation of the P-R interval.

Blocks distal to the bundle of His are considered **intraventricular conduction defects** and manifest as changes in QRS morphology and/or QRS axis. Included in this category are **nonspecific intraventricular conduction defects (IVCD), bundle branch blocks (BBB),** and **hemiblocks** (blocks of either the anterior or posterior fascicle of the left bundle branch).

A block in the left or right bundle branch creates a delay of the electrical impulse to its respective side while normal rapid conduction proceeds to the unblocked side. After the ventricle of the unblocked side depolarizes, conduction proceeds through the intraventricular septum to the ventricle on the side of the block. Therefore, in bundle branch block **(BBB)**, one ventricle fires slightly later than the other (rather than simultaneously). This causes two asynchronous superimposed QRS complexes. QRS widening results and an RR' pattern is usually produced (see EKG p. 73).

Recall that the left bundle splits into an anterior and posterior fascicle. A block in one of the fascicles (a hemiblock) will cause changes in the direction and timing of depolarization forces and hence characteristic EKG changes. Most notably, anterior hemiblock causes profound left axis deviation and posterior hemiblock causes profound right axis deviation. To understand the EKG changes more completely, it is helpful to realize that the anterior fascicle has an anterosuperior distribution and the posterior fascicle has a posteroinferior distribution. There are rich anastomoses between the two fascicles and this fact contributes to the lack of QRS widening seen in hemiblocks (in contradistinction to bundle branch blocks).

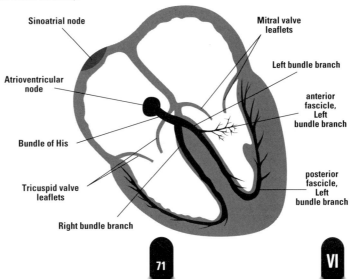

71

VI

Blocks

Right Bundle Branch Block (RBBB) - *(see diagram p. 76)*
EKG Findings

-Wide QRS complex (≥0.12 sec.).

-Terminal broad S wave in lead I.

-"M-shaped" QRS in right precordial leads (especially V1). This pattern is labelled RSR'. In RBBB the first R is usually smaller and the pattern is therefore designated rSR'.

-QRS is predominately positive in V1.

-Secondary repolarization changes present in some leads (S-T depression and T wave inversion that is in the opposite direction of the terminal deflection of the QRS).

-EKG diagnosis of RVH is not valid when RBBB exists.

-"Incomplete RBBB" exists when RBBB pattern is present but QRS duration is ≥0.10 and <0.12 sec. (some authors refer to this as "right intraventricular conduction defect").

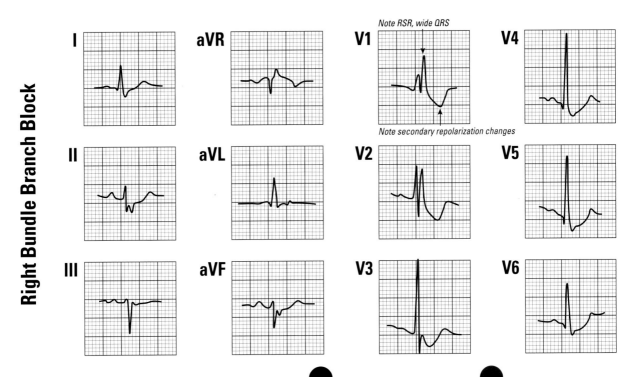

Right Bundle Branch Block

Note RSR, wide QRS

Note secondary repolarization changes

VI

Blocks

Left Bundle Branch Block (LBBB) - *(see diagram p. 77)*
EKG Findings

-Wide QRS complex (≥0.12 sec.).

-Absence of septal Q waves in I, aVL, V5, V6.

-"M-shaped" QRS in left precordial leads if present. This pattern is not seen as commonly as in RBBB and is usually less prominent.

-Secondary repolarization changes present in some leads (S-T depression and T wave inversion that is in the opposite direction of the terminal deflection of the QRS). Leads most likely effected are I, aVL, V5, V6.

-"Incomplete LBBB" exists when LBBB pattern is present but QRS duration is >0.10 and <0.12 sec. (some authors refer to this as "left intraventricular conduction defect").

-Diagnosis of MI is extremely difficult when LBBB exists. LBBB may cause Q waves, QS complexes, and ST-T changes that mimic and mask MI findings. Serial EKGs and clinical correlation will aid in diagnosis.

Left Bundle Branch Block

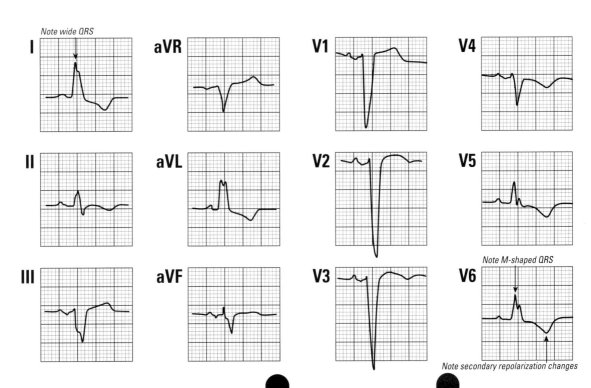

Note wide QRS

I   **aVR**   **V1**   **V4**

II   **aVL**   **V2**   **V5**

III   **aVF**   **V3**   **V6**

Note M-shaped QRS

Note secondary repolarization changes

VI

Right Bundle Branch Block (see p. 72)

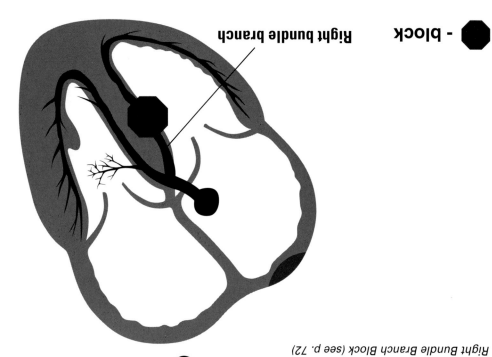

Right bundle branch

⬢ - **block**

Left Bundle Branch Block (see p. 74)

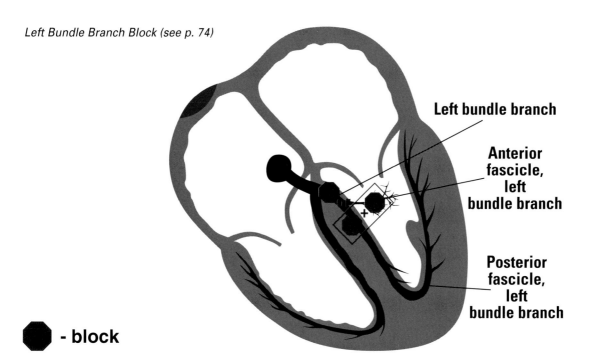

Left bundle branch

Anterior fascicle, left bundle branch

Posterior fascicle, left bundle branch

● - **block**

Left Anterior Fascicular Block

When the anterior fascicle is blocked, initial depolarization proceeds normally to the RV and posterior-inferior portion of the LV and is relatively unopposed by depolarizing forces heading towards the anterior-superior portion of the LV. Because these initial forces are moving away from the positive electrodes of leads I and aVL, and toward the positive electrodes of leads II, III, and aVF, the initial deflections of the QRS are often small Q waves in leads I and aVL, and small R waves in leads II, III and aVF. Subsequently, the remainder of the LV myocardium is depolarized in a leftward anterior-superior direction. These relatively unopposed depolarization forces are responsible for increased QRS voltage and left axis deviation.

EKG Findings

*-**Left Axis Deviation** of at least -45°.*
-Normal QRS duration
  (unless RBBB also present).
—The above criteria are essential.
The following may also occur.
  -Initial small Q waves in leads I, aVL.
  -Initial small R waves in leads II, III, aVF.
  -Increased QRS voltage in limb leads.

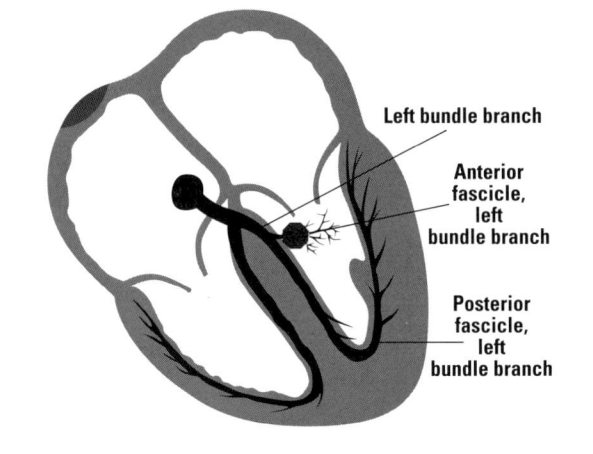

Left bundle branch

Anterior
fascicle,
left
bundle branch

Posterior
fascicle,
left
bundle branch

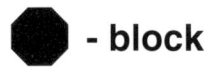 - block

Left Anterior Fascicular Block

Note the left axis deviation (see p. 20)

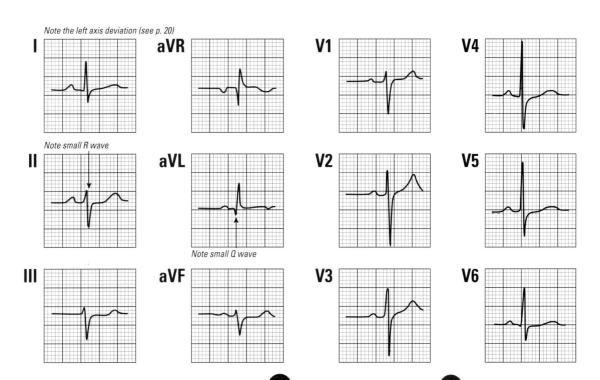

Note small R wave

Note small Q wave

I   aVR   V1   V4
II   aVL   V2   V5
III   aVF   V3   V6

VI

Blocks

Left Posterior Fascicular Block

When the posterior fascicle is blocked, initial depolarization moves in an anterior-superior direction (generally towards the positive electrodes of leads I, aVL and away from those of leads II, III, and aVF) hence the lead pattern of initial small Q and R waves is the reverse of that seen in left anterior hemiblock. An analogous right axis deviation then occurs as the remainder of the LV mass is depolarized in a rightward posterior-inferior direction.

EKG Findings

-**Right Axis Deviation** of at least +120°.
It is important to rule out other more
common causes of RAD such as RVH,
emphysema, lateral wall MI.

-Normal QRS duration
(unless RBBB also present).

—The above criteria are essential.
The following may also occur.

-Initial small R waves in leads I, aVL.
-Initial small Q waves in leads II, III, aVF.
-Increased QRS voltage in limb leads.

Left Posterior Fascicular Block

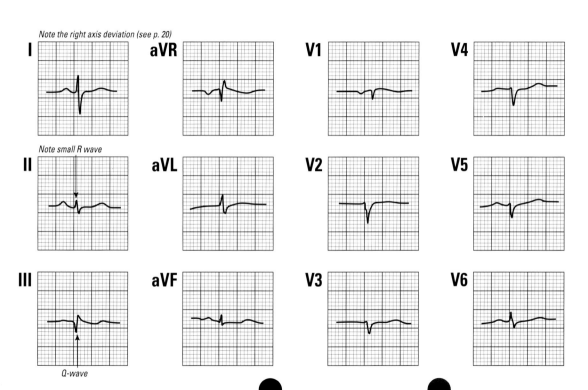

Note the right axis deviation (see p. 20)

I   aVR   V1   V4

Note small R wave

II   aVL   V2   V5

III   aVF   V3   V6

Q-wave

VI

Blocks

Bifascicular Block

Bifascicular Block is a conduction defect in two of the three peripheral major conduction fascicles of the Purkinje system (right bundle branch, left anterior fascicle, left posterior fascicle). Technically, therefore, LBBB can be considered in this category because it represents a functional (and sometimes anatomical block) of the anterior and posterior fascicles. However the term is more often reserved for a combination of RBBB and the simultaneous block of either the anterior or posterior fascicle of the left bundle branch. We encourage employment of the latter definition.

EKG Findings

-RBBB (p. 72) + left anterior fascicular block
(p. 78); or:
-RBBB (p. 72) + left posterior fascicular block
(p. 80).

Bifascicular Block

Note Axis deviation and changes associated with anterior fascicular block (see p. 78)

I aVR V1 V4

II aVL V2 V5

Note M-pattern of right bundle branch block

III aVF V3 V6

83

VI

Blocks

Trifascicular Block

Different authors present various concepts of trifascicular block. In its broadest definition it encompasses simultaneous blocks (complete or incomplete) of any three of the five ventricular conducting fascicles (His bundle, right bundle branch, left bundle branch, anterior and posterior fascicles of left bundle branch). When used in this vein it is merely a label applied to various combinations of intraventricular conduction defects and does not represent a specific clinical entity (hence constituting a laborious exercise in semantics). Block of the three peripheral fascicles (right bundle branch, left anterior and left posterior fascicles) resulting in **complete heart block** is a more specific and commonly used definition of trifascicular block. The resulting rhythm will be essentially the same as **third-degree AV block** (complete block of the AV node) (p. 216) although there is a technical anatomic difference between the two. Some authors accept a first-degree block as one of the three blocks necessary to diagnose a trifascicular block.

EKG Findings

-P waves are not conducted to ventricles. Independent pacemakers drive atrial and ventricular depolarization. Ventricular rate should be slower (reflecting ventricular escape). QRS complexes should be wide due to ventricular origin.

-Trifascicular block is identified when the patient is alternating between bifascicular block and complete heart block (pp. 82, 216).

Third-Degree Block

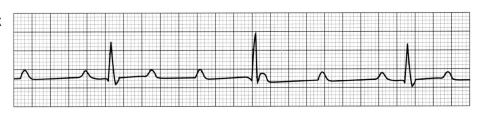

Drug Effects

QUINIDINE: Quinidine Effect

This antiarrhythmic drug has a vagolytic effect and slows conduction through the myocardium. Most of the EKG manifestations of the drug are, therefore, prolongations of various portions of the cardiac cycle.

EKG Findings

-Prolonged Q-T interval is the "hallmark," and earliest manifestation.

-Recall that Q-T interval must be corrected for age, sex, heart rate.

—These findings may also be present:

-U wave.

-S-T segment depression.

-Wide T wave.

-Wide, notched P wave.

-Torsade de Pointe (p.192).

-QRS prolongation.

Quinidine Effect

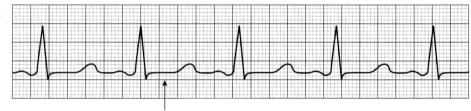

Note prolonged Q-T interval (see p. 8)

VII

Drug Effects

QUINIDINE: Quinidine Toxicity

The EKG manifestations are generally exaggerations of the effects seen when the drug is present in nontoxic levels. Prolongation of the QRS and Q-T interval by >25% may be early findings in toxicity.

EKG Findings

—One or more of the following may occur:

-Prolongation of corrected Q-T interval by > 25%.

-Sinus arrest.

-Atrial asystole.

-Prolonged P-R interval.

-Diffuse intraventricular block.

-Widening of QRS.

-Ventricular fibrillation.

-Ventricular ectopy.

-Torsade de Pointe.

Miscellaneous Drugs that Prolong Q-T Interval

Several drugs (in addition to Quinidine) are known to prolong the Q-T interval in nontoxic levels. Among the most common are:

> Procainamide
> Disopyramide
> Phenothiazines
> Tricyclic antidepressants
> Other antiarrhythmics

Drug Effects

DIGITALIS: Digitalis Effect

Note: Digitalis effect is an EKG change commonly seen in patients on digitalis, and does not necessarily imply toxicity.

EKG Findings

-S-T segment depression (in leads with predominately positive QRS) which usually has a "U" shaped configuration. See figure on next page.
-T wave flattening and inversion.
-Prolongation of P-R interval.
-Shortening of Q-T interval .

Digitalis Effect

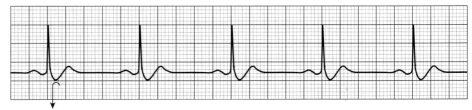

Note appearance of a "hook tugging down" the S-T segment

DIGITALIS: Digitalis Toxicity

80% to 90% of patients with digitalis toxicity will experience cardiac dysrhythmias.

EKG Findings

-Many different cardiac dysrhythmias are possible with digitalis toxicity. Considering the actions of digitalis (decreased automaticity of SA node, decreased conduction through AV nodal tissue, increased automaticity of AV nodal and other ectopic pacemakers) certain dysrhythmias are predictably more likely to occur than others. For example, one would expect to see ventricular ectopy and it is, in fact, one of the most common signs of digitalis excess. Rather than providing an exhaustive list of the possible dysrhythmias, we will caution the reader to suspect the diagnosis whenever a patient using a digitalis preparation develops complex dysrhythmias. There are, however, a few dysrhythmias that are considered "classic."

DIGITALIS: Digitalis Toxicity (cont.)

—Classic Dysrhythmias:
-PAT with variable AV block.
-High-grade AV block.
-Bidirectional ventricular tachycardia (wide ventricular complexes alternating in polarity).

—Common Dysrhythmias:
-PVCs.
-Ventricular bigeminy (especially multifocal). This is one of the "hallmarks."
-Junctional rhythm.
-Nonparoxysmal junctional tachycardia.

Digitalis and Quinidine (Combined Effects)

EKG Findings
-This combination may closely resemble hypokalemia (see p. 94).

Electrolytes

POTASSIUM (K+)

Recognition of EKG manifestations of potassium imbalance can be made easier by use of the phrase: <u>Potassium lives under the T wave</u>. No electrophysiological phenomenon is suggested by this phrase. It is merely intended to provide visualization to enhance memory. In hypokalemia, one can visualize that there is not enough K+ to "hold up the T wave," so it flattens. In hyperkalemia, the abundance of K+ causes a tenting of the T wave. As the K+ continues to rise—this tenting progressively pulls on the rest of the EKG tracing— making the QRS wider, lengthening the P-R interval, and diminishing the height of the P wave.

POTASSIUM: Hypokalemia

A variety of ST-T abnormalities may occur when the serum potassium is below normal. Following is a list of EKG findings that suggest this diagnosis.

EKG Findings

-Flattening of T wave and development of prominent U wave (U≥T). These are considered the earliest and most common findings. Best leads for examination of U waves are V2-V4.

-S-T segment depression. CAUTION: Consider other causes (p. 44).

-T wave inversion.

-Q-T interval is usually of normal duration. Merging of T and U waves may appear as a late T wave and therefore make the Q-T interval appear prolonged.

-Increase in height and width of P wave, especially in II, III, aVF. This pattern is designated "pseudo-P-pulmonale." These P wave changes are usually later manifestations.

Hypokalemia

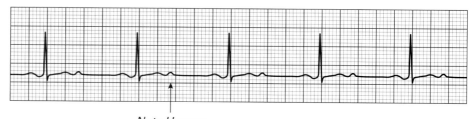

Note U wave

Electrolytes

POTASSIUM: Hyperkalemia

EKG Findings

-T wave tenting (tall, narrow symmetrically high-peaked T waves). This T wave change is the earliest manifestation.

—As K+ continues to increase:

-T wave height increases.

-Prolongation of P-R interval.

-Shortening of Q-T interval.

-Diminution of P wave height. P waves may disappear completely—representing atrial arrest. SA node is still pacing but depolarization is sent to AV node via conduction pathways while atria fail to depolarize.

-QRS widening [which may represent Intraventricular conduction defect (IVCD)].

-Upsloping S-T segment depression.

—As K+ continues to increase:

-QRS progressively widens—**sine wave appearance** may develop—followed by **Ventricular Fibrillation** and **Asystole**.

Hyperkalemia

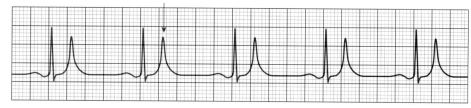

Note T wave tenting

Electrolytes

CALCIUM (Ca2+)

Recall that the influx of calcium through slow channels is responsible for the plateau phase of depolarization (phase II) of the myocardial cell. With this in mind, one can visualize that an optimal level of extracellular calcium is necessary to provide the proper gradient to drive the normal rate of this influx. A normal rate of influx is necessary for normal timing of the depolarization/repolarization cycle of the cell. Therefore, the cycle is prolonged in states of low calcium availability and the cycle is shortened in states of high calcium availability in the extracellular fluid.

CALCIUM: Hypocalcemia

EKG Findings

-Prolongation of Q-T interval due to S-T segment prolongation. (Recall that the Q-T interval varies with age, sex, and heart rate) (p. 7).

-T waves are usually normal, but may become inverted in cases of profound hypocalcemia.

$$Q\text{-}Tc = \frac{Q\text{-}T}{\sqrt{R\text{-}R \ Interval}}$$

A normal Q-Tc interval is approximately 0.44±0.02 second

Hypocalcemia

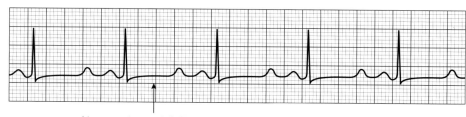

Note prolonged Q-T interval

VIII

Electrolytes

CALCIUM: Hypercalcemia

EKG Findings
-Shortening of Q-T interval. (Recall that the Q-T interval varies with age, sex, and heart rate) (p. 8).

$$Q\text{-}Tc = \frac{Q\text{-}T}{\sqrt{R\text{-}R\ Interval}}$$

A normal Q-Tc interval is approximately 0.44±0.02 second

Hypercalcemia

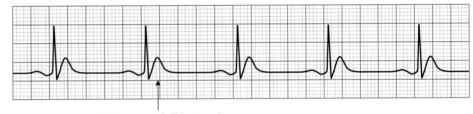

Note short Q-T interval

VIII

Pericarditis

Pericarditis is an inflammation of the pericardial sac. Etiologies include viral, bacterial, MI, collagen vascular diseases, uremia, and metastases. As the inflamed pericardium contacts the epicardial surface, ST-T changes resembling the current of injury pattern associated with myocardial injury/infarction develop. Differentiation of pericarditis from myocardial injury/ischemia is based on the more diffuse nature of pericarditis. The inflamed pericardium contacts the majority of the heart—hence the changes are more likely throughout the EKG. Recall that MI is a relatively local phenomenon corresponding to the location of occluded coronary circulation and that lead-specific EKG changes occur (see MI p. 124).

EKG Findings

-Characteristic S-T segment elevation which is flat or has an upward concavity.

-Elevation of T wave from the baseline.

—The combination of these ST-T changes and a preceding positive QRS result in a configuration resembling a "*Fireman's Hat*" (note V5 and V6 on following page). These changes may be widespread and should include anterior and inferior leads. This configuration may be present in all leads except aVR which will often show S-T segment depression.

-No significant Q waves will be present. If they are, MI must be considered. Pericarditis alone will not cause Q waves. It is possible to have MI and pericarditis concurrently.

-T wave inversion may be a late finding.

-Low voltage will be the predominant EKG finding if a large pericardial effusion is associated with the pericarditis.

Pericarditis

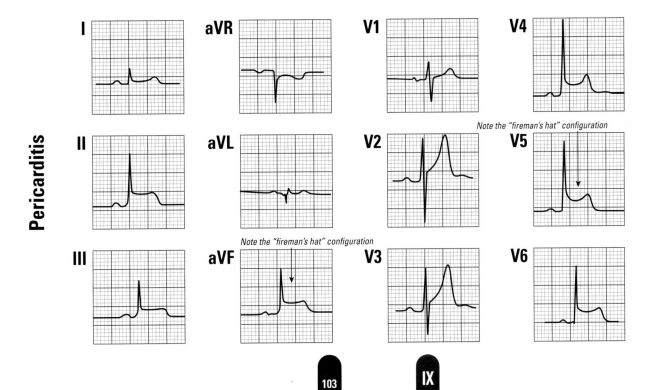

I aVR V1 V4

Note the "fireman's hat" configuration

II aVL V2 V5

Note the "fireman's hat" configuration

III aVF V3 V6

Miscellaneous Disorders

Hypothermia

Decreasing body temperature causes vagal effects, slowing of the depolarization/repolarization process, ionic shifts, irritability, and slowed conduction. The resultant EKG manifestations will revert to normal if body temperature is normalized. Dysrhythmias, including ventricular fibrillation, are common during rewarming.

EKG Findings
-Bradycardia (usually sinus).
-Prolongation of all intervals (P-R, QRS, Q-T).
-Atrial fibrillation or flutter.
-J wave (also called O wave or Osborn wave). This is a pointed elevation of the initial portion of the S-T segment at the J-point. Best seen in limb and left chest leads. See figure below.
-T wave flattening (due to hypokalemia as K+ shifts into cells).
—The above signs should alert one to the diagnosis of hypothermia. As temperature continues to drop, the following may occur:
-Ventricular ectopy.
-Various conduction blocks.
-Ventricular fibrillation.
-Asystole.

Hypothermia

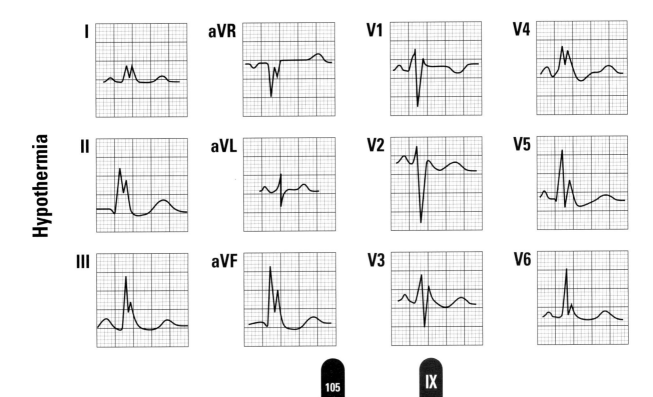

I   aVR   V1   V4

II   aVL   V2   V5

III   aVF   V3   V6

105   IX

Ventricular Aneurysm

A ventricular aneurysm is a dyskinetic segment of myocardium which may be the result of infarct. This segment of the ventricular wall bulges out when the remainder of the ventricle contracts. The diagnosis should be suspected when a fully evolved transmural myocardial infarction pattern persists for greater than 3 months. EKG is not extremely sensitive for ventricular aneurysm.

EKG Findings

-Persistent current of injury pattern (S-T segment elevation). Q waves and inverted T waves may persist also.

Ventricular Aneurysm

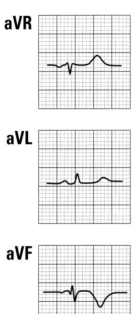

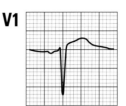

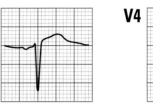

Note S-T elevation, Q wave, and inverted T wave

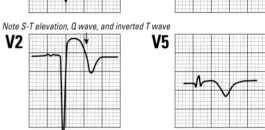

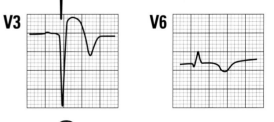

I aVR V1 V4

II aVL V2 V5

III aVF V3 V6

Pulmonary Embolism (PE)

Pulmonary embolism is an acute respiratory compromise that occurs when a pulmonary artery or one of its branches is occluded by a lodged embolus. The occlusion causes a sudden increase in pulmonary circuit resistance. Most of the EKG manifestations reflect acute changes in the right heart that are secondary to backpressure from the increased resistance. For example, acute right ventricular dilatation would be expected and it is sometimes demonstrated by right axis shift and right ventricular strain pattern. Furthermore, right atrial dilatation may ensue and be evident by a P-pulmonale pattern (p. 56).

The EKG is not particularly sensitive for PE, and should be used in conjunction with other diagnostic modalities.

Acute Cor Pulmonale is the clinical entity said to exist when a PE (or some other acute respiratory condition) causes pathologic changes in the heart and hence EKG changes. When present, the EKG changes usually evolve rapidly (within minutes) and resolve in hours to days. EKG changes are variable, and some combination of the features listed on the following page may be seen.

Chronic Cor Pulmonale is a condition characterized by increased resistance in the pulmonary circuit. This increased resistance causes a compensatory hypertrophy of the right ventricle. RAE and right heart failure may develop as the disease progresses. An acute form of the disease occurs with dilatation of the right ventricle associated with right heart failure in response to an acute increase in pulmonary resistance. This occurs in pulmonary embolism.

Pulmonary Embolus (cont.)

EKG Findings

-Sinus tachycardia (almost always present).

-Right axis deviation.

-P-pulmonale (P wave height ≥ 2.5 mm in one or more of leads II, III, aVF) (See Right Atrial Enlargement, p. 56).

-Inverted T waves in right chest leads (V1-V3) indicating "Right Ventricular Strain" (see p. 61).

-Pseudo-diaphragmatic (inferior wall) myocardial ischemia or infarction pattern. This presentation usually consists of significant Q wave, S-T elevation, and T wave inversion in lead III. Lead II will not show this pattern and is more likely to show a deep S wave. This difference as well as the absence of a Q wave in aVF helps distinguish pulmonary embolus from inferior wall myocardial infarction.

Pulmonary Embolus (cont.)

EKG Findings

-S1, Q3, T3 pattern. The pattern consists of an S wave in lead I, a significant Q wave in III and an inverted T wave in III.

-S1, S2, S3 pattern. The pattern consists of prominent S waves in leads I, II, III.

-Prominent S waves in V5, V6.

-Complete or incomplete RBBB of acute onset. It is usually transient.

-Diffuse ST-T changes, especially in right chest leads.

Miscellaneous Disorders

Wolff-Parkinson-White Syndrome (WPW)

This syndrome consists of premature activation ("preexcitation") of a portion of the ventricular myocardium. The impulse is carried to a portion of the ventricle by AV bypass tracts that form direct connections between the atria and the ventricles. The EKG corollary of these bypass tracts is represented by shortening of the PR interval and slurring of the upstroke (<u>delta wave</u>) and prolongation of the QRS. The QRS represents a fusion complex resulting from dual activation of the bypass tract and the normal AV conduction system. Patients with WPW have a propensity to develop supraventricular macro-reentry tachyarrhythmias and possibly atrial fibrillation, which can result in ventricular fibrillation. It is important to identify WPW because pharmacological therapy is different for paroxysmal supraventricular tachycardia (PSVT) when preexcitation is present. The treatment of choice for WPW is radiofrequency ablation.

EKG Findings
—*These findings may be present in several leads.*
-*Delta wave (may be subtle).*
-*Short P-R interval (≤0.12 seconds).*
-*Prolonged QRS (≥0.10 seconds).*

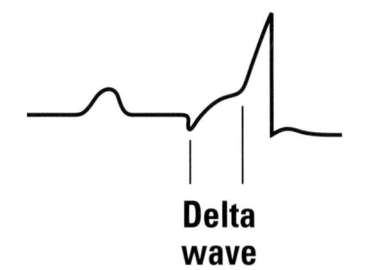

Delta wave

Wolf-Parkinson-White Syndrome (WPW)

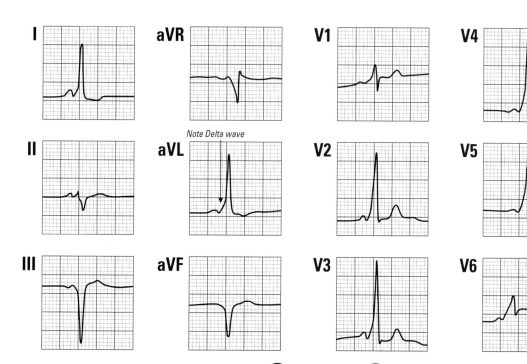

Note Delta wave

113 IX

Miscellaneous Disorders

Lown-Ganong-Levine Syndrome (LGL)

LGL syndrome is preexcitation demonstrated by a short P-R interval but a normal QRS and no delta wave (p. 112). The pattern in some patients is thought to represent rapid conduction from the atria to the AV junction (bypassing the normal delay of the AV node) via an accessory tract (James fibers). Patients with LGL experience a higher incidence of dysrhythmias, especially paroxysmal atrial tachycardia (PAT).

EKG Findings

-Short P-R interval (all leads).
-No delta wave is present.
-Intermittent supraventricular tachyarrhythmias.

} *All three are required to diagnose this syndrome.*

Lown-Ganong-Levine Syndrome (LGL)

Note short P-R interval and lack of a delta wave

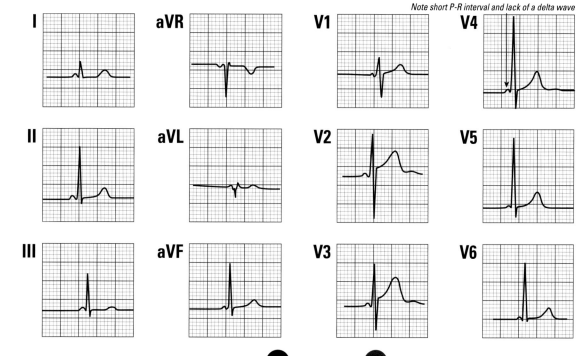

115

IX

Subarachnoid Hemorrhage/Cerebrovascular Accident (CVA)

A CVA may cause EKG changes, especially when it is accompanied by a subarachnoid hemorrhage. One would not obtain an EKG for the specific purpose of making such a diagnosis; however, the EKG is indicated to aid in the evaluation of cardiac status of an acutely decompensating patient. Most prominent among the findings listed below are deeply inverted, wide T waves with a diffuse distribution (sometimes referred to as "CVA-T wave pattern"). The EKG findings are thought to reflect changes in the autonomic nervous system rather than pathology of the myocardium. Less frequently, other central nervous system disorders have been implicated to produce similar EKG changes. Included among them are brain tumors, heat stroke, head trauma, delirium tremens, diabetic coma, and hepatic coma.

EKG Findings

-Deeply inverted, wide T waves with diffuse distribution.
-Nonspecific ST-T changes.
-Prolonged Q-T interval (remember to correct for age, sex, heart rate) (p. 8).
-Prominent U waves.
-Supraventricular tachycardia.

Subarachnoid hemorrhage/ Cerebrovascular accident

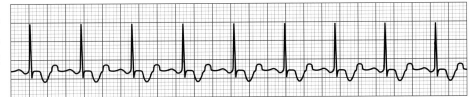

Repolarization Variant

A normal variant of S-T segment elevation has been characterized. It most frequently occurs in young, healthy men (especially blacks). It has been called "Early Repolarization" but this term is a misnomer. It has also been called "Juvenile Precordial Pattern." The elevation ranges from slight to prominent (up to 4 mm) and is most often present in some or all of the precordial leads. The S-T segment may fall to baseline during exercise or isoproterenol administration. The pattern is stable over time and reciprocal S-T segment depression does not occur (except perhaps in aVR). These findings, along with clinical correlation, help distinguish repolarization variant from acute MI and acute pericarditis.

EKG Findings

-S-T segment elevation in some or all of the precordial leads. There is usually a notch during the descent of the R wave prior to formation of the S-T segment and the T wave usually appears as a distinct wave form rather than being slurred with the S-T segment.

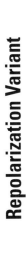

Repolarization Variant

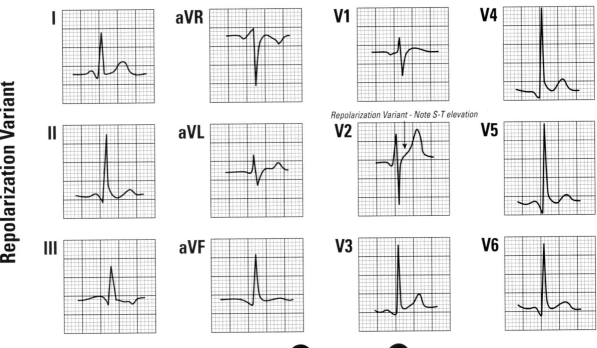

I   aVR   V1   V4

Repolarization Variant - Note S-T elevation

II   aVL   V2   V5

III   aVF   V3   V6

Ischemia, Injury, and Infarction

Ischemia can be transient without causing damage, or it may progress to injury and infarction (necrosis). Due to the high pressure on the subendocardium exerted by the adjacent high pressure in the ventricular chamber, ischemic heart disease tends to begin in the subendocardial layer and progress to the subepicardial layer. Ischemia, injury and infarction affect the electrical properties of the myocardial cells, and therefore can cause alterations in the EKG during the QRS complex, S-T segment and T wave (ventricular depolarization and repolarization). Following are summaries of the EKG changes diagnostic of ischemia, injury and infarction.

Ischemia

This is the earliest result of inadequate blood supply to the myocardium, and if the the blood supply is restored, is reversible.

EKG Findings

-*Symmetric T wave inversion (This represents subendocardial involvement).*
-*S-T segment depression (This also represents subendocardial involvement). This is the most common manifestation of ischemia.*
Note: *S-T segment elevation rarely can be representative of transmyocardial ischemia without injury. It may represent ischemia in atypical angina (also known as variant angina and Prinzmetal's angina).*
-*U wave inversion (if U wave is present).*
-*Tall, peaked "hyperacute" T waves may be an early sign of ischemia.*

Ischemia

Note T wave inversion

121   X

Ischemia, Injury, and Infarction

Injury

This is a more severe or sustained loss of blood supply to the myocardium, but is still reversible if blood supply can be restored.

EKG Findings

-S-T segment elevation. The S-T segment should be elevated >1 mm above the baseline. This is known as the "current of injury." The S-T segment can have variable shapes.

-May see tall, peaked "hyperacute" T waves.

-T wave inversion.

Injury

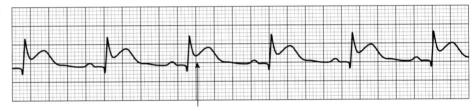

Note S-T segment elevation

Infarction

Irreversible structural changes in the myocardium from severe or sustained loss of blood supply.

EKG Findings

-Significant Q waves (>1mm wide or >25% of R wave height). Significant Q waves are the most definitive EKG evidence of infarction.

-S-T segment and T wave changes as described for injury (in the absence of Q waves) are suggestive but not definitive for infarction (p. 122).

-Reciprocal Changes:

Q waves, S-T segment elevation, and inverted T waves that occur in leads that represent the region of infarction are called **indicative changes**. Additionally, **reciprocal changes** may occur in leads which represent the LV wall anatomically opposite the region of infarction. Reciprocal changes are usually of less magnitude than the indicative changes (p. 142).

EKG Findings Associated With Reciprocal Changes
(note especially leads I and aVL on following page)

-Increased height of R waves.

-S-T segment depression.

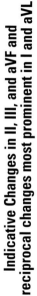

Indicative Changes in II, III, and aVF and reciprocal changes most prominent in I and aVL

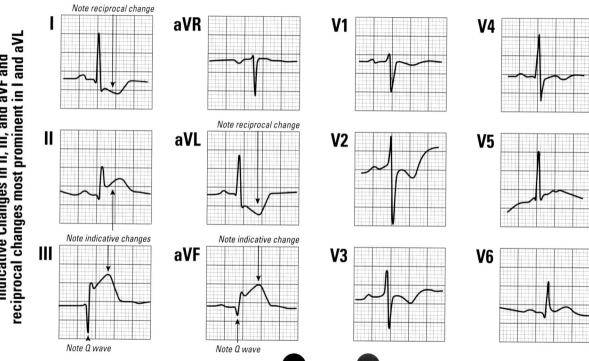

I — *Note reciprocal change*

aVR

V1

V4

II

aVL — *Note reciprocal change*

V2

V5

III — *Note indicative changes* / *Note Q wave*

aVF — *Note indicative change* / *Note Q wave*

V3

V6

125

X

The evolution of Q wave Infarction

It is an important concept that the EKG stages of infarction occur not all at once, but in stages. These stages are listed below and illustrated below diagrammatically. The stages presented here are considered typical, but keep in mind that much variability exists in the time course of such EKG changes.

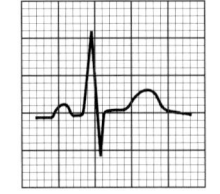

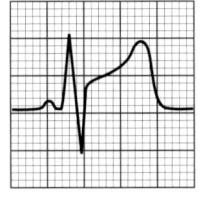

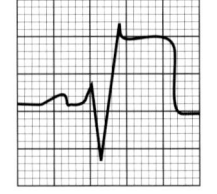

1. Before occlusion of the coronary artery. Normal electrocardiogram.

2. Within several hours after occlusion. Injury of the subendocardium and ischemia of the myocardium. Note the normal R wave, the early S-T segment elevation and the peaked T wave.

3. 24 hours after occlusion. Ischemia and injury of the myocardium. Early necrosis of the endocardium. Note the decreased height of the R wave and the increased elevation of the S-T segment.

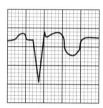

4. One to three days after occlusion.
Myocardial necrosis: completion of a transmural infarction. Note the formation of a significant Q wave (QS in this case), the near loss of the R wave, the inversion of the T wave, and the decreasing elevation of the S-T segment.

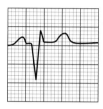

5. Two weeks to two months after occlusion. Infarcted area has now been replaced by fibrous tissue. Note that the Q wave usually is permanent, and that some of the R wave height may be regained. The T wave has returned to its upright position.

X

The Diagnosis of Infarction in patients with bundle branch blocks (see also p. 70)

The EKG diagnosis of infarction is extremely difficult in patients who have left bundle branch block. Q waves, S-T segment elevation and T wave abnormalities are common findings in patients with left bundle branch block, and may cause an inappropriate diagnosis of infarction.

<u>Right bundle branch block</u>, however, does not generally interfere with the EKG diagnosis of infarction.

Non-Q WAVE INFARCTION

Persistent S-T segment depression or symmetrical T wave inversion in the absence of Q waves may represent infarction. The EKG tracing may be identical to an ischemic pattern. Therefore, the diagnosis of subendocardial infarction relies upon other additional data (clinical course, laboratory data).

Myocardial Ischemia

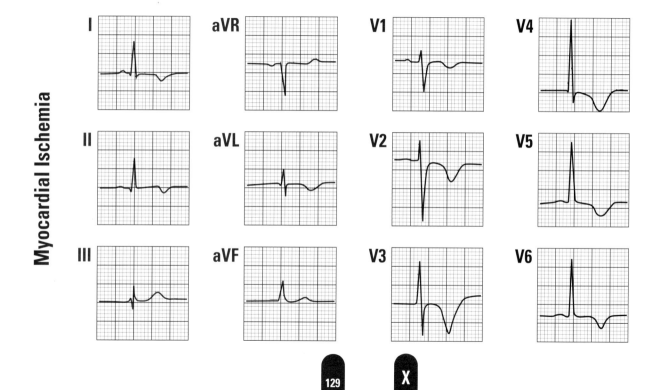

I aVR V1 V4

II aVL V2 V5

III aVF V3 V6

129 X

The Evolution of Non-Q wave Infarction

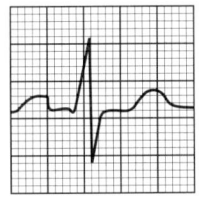

1. Before infarction. Normal electro-cardiogram.

S-T Depression   S-T Elevation

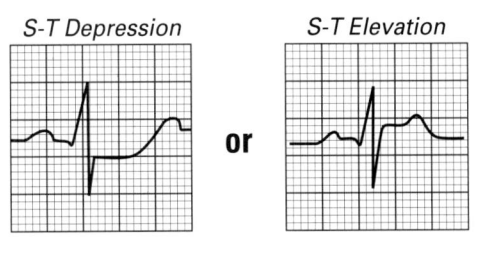

or

2. Several hours after arterial compromise. Ischemia and injury of the subendocardial muscle have occurred. Note that the S-T segment can either be elevated or depressed.

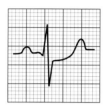

3. Two days after arterial compromise. Non-Q wave infarction, confirmed by elevation in cardiac enzymes, has occurred. Note the absence of a significant Q wave. T wave inversion may or may not occur.

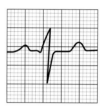

4. Two months after infarction. The electrocardiogram has returned to normal. If T wave inversion occurred during infarction, it may persist.

Infarction (cont.)

Once it has been determined that EKG changes associated with ischemia, injury, or infarction are present, an analysis of the 12 lead EKG can often suggest the area of the left ventricle that is involved. The left ventricle is divided into four areas: anterior, lateral, inferior (also referred to as diaphragmatic), and posterior. Leads placed over these areas are grouped together to form a basis for localizing the area that is undergoing vascular compromise. It is important to understand that in clinical situations, the changes of injury, ischemia and infarction may be seen in only some, or in all of the leads listed under "EKG findings." It is even possible to have myocardial infarction with a normal electrocardiogram.

Potential Areas of Left Ventricular Infarction

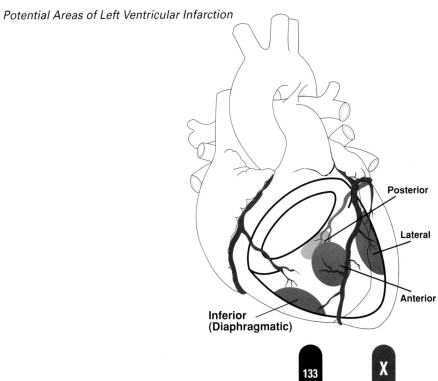

Posterior

Lateral

Anterior

Inferior (Diaphragmatic)

Ischemia, Injury, and Infarction

Infarction (cont.)
Anterior Wall

Ischemia, injury and infarction of the anterior wall are common, and are clinically very important since the pathways of conduction are often affected.

EKG Findings

-Evidence of ischemia, injury or infarction (p. 120) in leads **V1-V6, I,**
    and **aVL.**

-Poor R wave progression. The R wave normally increases gradually
    in height from **V1** through **V3** or **V4**. A loss or reversal of this
    normal progression may indicate anterior myocardial infarction.

-In the case of anterior myocardial infarction, grouping with other
    types of infarction is sometimes used. This is illustrated as follows:

        -**Anteroseptal infarction**: changes associated with infarction in
          V1-V4.

        -**Anterolateral infarction**: changes associated with infarction in
          V2-V6. The inclusion of **V5** and **V6** implies lateral wall involve
          ment. Involvement of **leads I** and **aVL** may also occur in
          anterolateral infarction.

        -**Extensive anterior infarction**: when changes associated with
          infarction are seen in **leads I, aVL,** and **V1-V6,** the term
          "extensive anterior myocardial infarction" may be used.

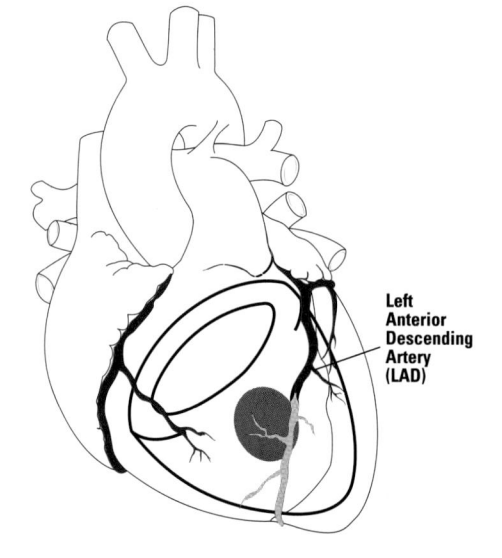

Left
Anterior
Descending
Artery
(LAD)

Anterior Wall Myocardial Infarction

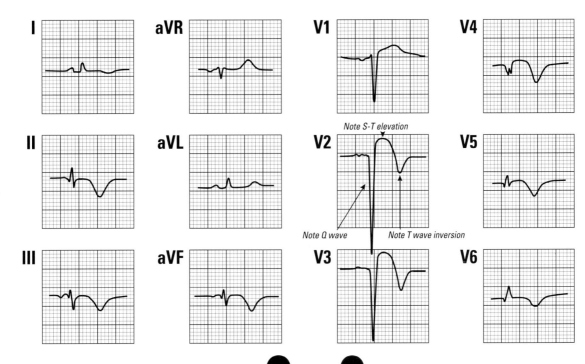

I

aVR

V1

V4

II

aVL

V2

Note S-T elevation

V5

Note Q wave   Note T wave inversion

III

aVF

V3

V6

135   X

Infarction (cont.)
Lateral Wall

Ischemic changes may involve the lateral wall alone, or may be in combination with other areas of the ventricle.

EKG Findings

-Evidence of ischemia, injury or infarction (p. 120) in **leads I, aVL, V5, and V6**.

-In the case of lateral myocardial infarction, grouping with other types of infarction is sometimes used. This is illustrated as follows:

-**Anterolateral infarction**: changes associated with infarction in **leads V2-V6, I, and aVL**.

-**Inferolateral infarction**: changes associated with infarction in **leads II, III, and aVF** along with **leads V5 and V6**.

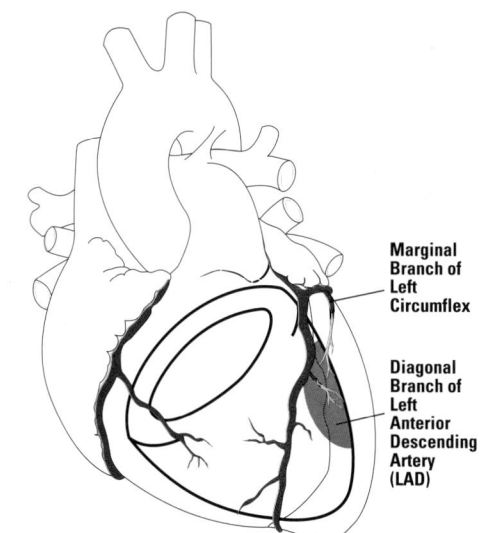

Marginal Branch of Left Circumflex

Diagonal Branch of Left Anterior Descending Artery (LAD)

Lateral Wall Infarction

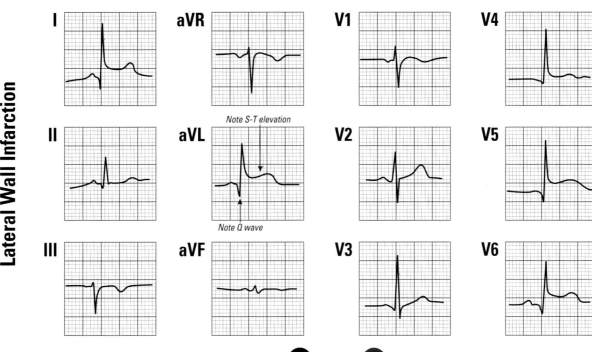

I

aVR

V1

V4

II

aVL

Note S-T elevation

Note Q wave

V2

V5

III

aVF

V3

V6

Infarction (cont.)
Inferior (Diaphragmatic) Wall

The inferior wall is a common area of ischemic involvement. Like anterior and lateral wall involvement, it often may involve the inferior wall alone, or may be in combination with other areas of the ventricle.

EKG Findings

-Evidence of ischemia, injury, or infarction (p. 120) in **leads II, III,** and **aVF.**

—**Note:** A prominent Q wave in lead III alone may be a normal finding. If Q waves are also seen in **leads II** and/or **aVF,** infarction is more likely.

-In the case of inferior wall myocardial infarction, grouping with other types of infarction is sometimes used. This is illustrated as follows:

-**Inferolateral infarction:** changes associated with infarction (p. 124) in **leads II, III, aVF, V5,** and **V6.**

-**Inferoposterior (inferobasal) infarction:** changes associated with infarction in **leads II, III, aVF,** along with a large R wave in **V1,** an upright T wave in **V1,** and a Q wave in **V6** (sometimes not a significant Q wave).

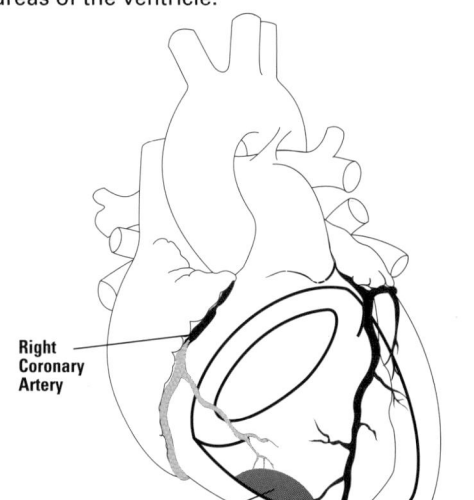

Right Coronary Artery

Inferior (Diaphragmatic)

Inferior Wall Myocardial Infarction

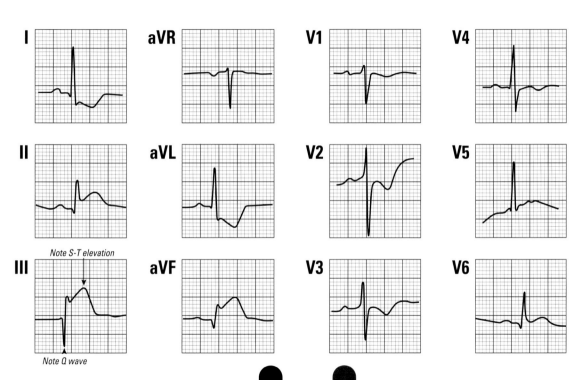

I

aVR

V1

V4

II

aVL

V2

V5

Note S-T elevation

III

aVF

V3

V6

Note Q wave

139

X

Ischemia, Injury, and Infarction

Infarction (cont.)
Posterior Wall

True posterior wall infarctions are not common because of the relatively small size of the posterior surface, and the excellent blood supply to this area. Because no leads overlie the posterior wall, diagnosis is based upon reciprocal changes in the chest leads.

EKG Findings (for posterior wall myocardial infarction)

-An unusually large R wave in **lead V1** (a reciprocal [mirror image] of a posterior wall Q wave).

> **—Note:** This can be difficult to differentiate from right ventricular hypertrophy. It is important as always to take into account the clinical situation. In addition, the presence or absence of right axis deviation may be helpful since RAD often occurs in RVH.

-An upright T wave in **V1** (a reciprocal (mirror image) of a posterior wall T wave inversion).

-Diagnosis of posterior infarction can be aided by placing leads on the back (posterior leads). These are not demonstrated on the EKG below.

-Often associated with inferior wall infarction.

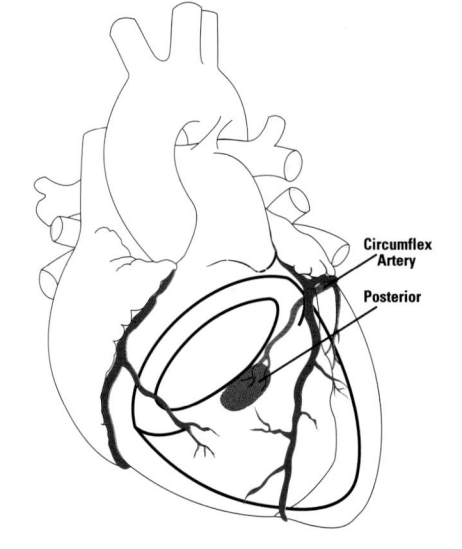

Circumflex Artery

Posterior

Posterior Wall Myocardial Infarction

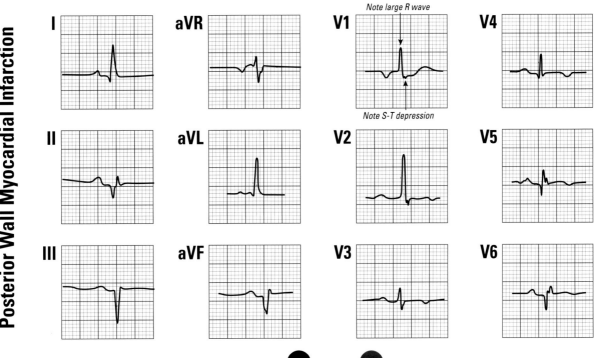

I   aVR   V1 *Note large R wave* / *Note S-T depression*   V4

II   aVL   V2   V5

III   aVF   V3   V6

Infarction (cont.)

Summary of indicative and reciprocal changes localizing infarction to region of LV and predominantly involved coronary vessels.

Portion of LV Wall	Leads of Indicative Change	Leads of Reciprocal Change
Inferior (right coronary artery)	**II, III, aVF**	**I, aVL, chest leads** (anterior leads)
Anterior (L anterior descending)	**I, aVL, V1-V6**	**II, III, aVF** (inferior leads)
Lateral (L circumflex)	**I, aVL, V5, V6**	**V1**
Posterior (distal branches of L circumflex or R coronary)	*no indicative changes*	**V1, V2**

Infarction (cont.)

Right Ventricle

Infarction of the right ventricle is more common than once believed. It is associated frequently with inferior (diaphragmatic) wall infarction. Accurate diagnosis relies upon a high index of suspicion, since special precordial leads placed on the right side of the chest must be used.

EKG Findings

-S-T segment elevation in leads V4R-V6R (anterior leads placed on the right side of the chest rather than the left side) (p. 17).

-May be associated with an inferior wall infarction (changes associated with infarction (p. 138) in leads II, III, and aVF).

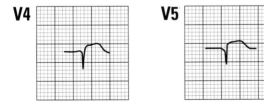

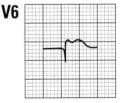

X

Sinus Tachycardia

Sinus tachycardia implies a rapid heart rate from an increase in the automaticity of the sinus node in response to physiologic stimuli. The electrical stimulus travels along the normal conduction pathways.

May be normal (esp. in children) or may be seen with:

Stress	Shock
Dehydration	Myocardial infarction (p. 124)
Digitalis toxicity (p. 92)	Hyperthyroidism
Pulmonary embolism (p. 108)	
Anemia	
Exercise	
Drug effects (i.e., atropine, epinephrine)	
Fever	
Pain	
Caffeine, nicotine, or alcohol ingestion	
Congestive heart failure	

EKG Findings
-Heart rate above 100 beats per minute.
-Normal P wave, QRS complex and T wave.
-P-R interval may be slightly shortened.

Sinus tachycardia
(rate 120)

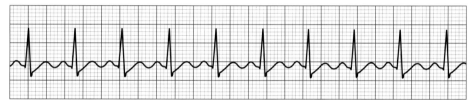

Sinus Bradycardia

Sinus bradycardia implies a decrease in automaticity of the sinus node resulting in a slow heart rate. This may be in response to conditioning or sleep.

May be seen with:

        During sleep
        Hypothyroidism
        Hyperkalemia (p. 96)
        Drug effects (e.g., beta-blockers)
        During endotracheal intubation
        Increased intracranial pressure
        Sick Sinus Syndrome
        Myocardial infarction (p. 124)
        With mechanical ventilation
        With increased vagal tone (e.g., athletes)

EKG Findings

        -Heart rate below 60 beats per minute.
        -Normal P wave, QRS complex, and T wave.

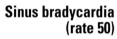**Sinus bradycardia**
(rate 50)

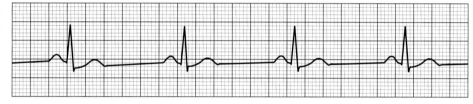

Sinus Arrhythmia

Sinus Arrhythmia is a cyclic variation in heart rate, usually associated with inspiration and expiration. The heart rate tends to increase during inspiration and decrease during expiration.

May also be seen in athletes or with:
> Increased intracranial pressure
> Sick Sinus Syndrome
> Digitalis toxicity (p. 92)
> Myocardial infarction (p. 124)
> Chronic lung disease

EKG Findings
> -Sinus rhythm.
> -Normal P wave, QRS complex, and T wave.
> -A variation of heart rate of about 10% associated with respiration (phasic sinus arrhythmia) or unassociated with respiration (nonphasic sinus arrhythmia).

Sinus arrhythmia

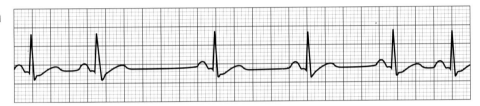

Sinoatrial block

Sinoatrial block occurs when impulses generated in the SA node are not conducted. SA block is manifested by dropped P waves. This mechanism is different from sinus arrest in which there is no impulse generated. If there is shortening of the P-P intervals leading to the dropped P wave, this is sometimes termed "SA Wenckebach." If the absent P wave is seen as an exact multiple of the other sinus cycles, "Type II" SA block is said to exist.

May be seen with:
> Sick Sinus Syndrome
> Digitalis Toxicity
> Quinidine Toxicity
> Increased vagal tone

Sinoatrial block (cont.)

EKG Findings

SA Wenckebach decreased P-P interval on successive beats, followed by loss of P wave and QRS complex. *(Note: this is contrast to Type I AV block where P-P intervals increase before dropped beat).*
-Type II: regular P-P interval with occasional dropped P wave and QRS complex.

Non conducted P waves

Sinoatrial block (type II)

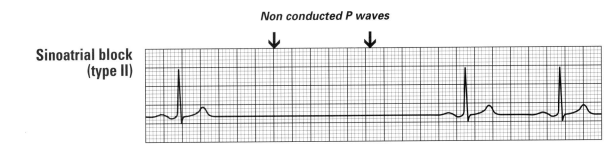

Sinus Arrest

Failure of impulse formation in sinus node.

EKG Findings

-Absence of P waves and QRS complex.
-Presence of escape beats after initial pause (p. 195).

Sinus arrest

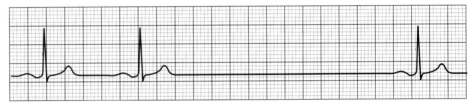

Premature Atrial Complexes (PAC)

PACs are premature ectopic atrial beats of non-sinus origin. The resultant deflection is called P' (P prime). The shape of the P' wave is dependent upon its location of origin. If the impulse originates in the area of the sinus node, the P' wave will look similar to the normal P wave with the exception of its being premature. If the impulse originates low in the atria, retrograde conduction to the SA node will result in an inverted P' wave in the inferior leads (II, III, aVF). When the SA node is depolarized, it resets itself and continues to fire at its inherent rate. Therefore, the P'-P interval will be the same as the normal P-P interval; this is termed an <u>incomplete compensatory pause</u>.

Causes of PACs include:
> Intake of caffeine or tobacco
> Digitalis toxicity (p. 92)
> Theophylline
> Hypokalemia (p. 94)
> Hypomagnesemia

EKG Findings
> -P' wave may appear different from normal P wave depending on location of origin.
> -Premature ectopic P wave (P' wave).
> -Incomplete compensatory pause.
> -Normal QRS complexes.

Normal sinus rhythm with premature atrial contractions

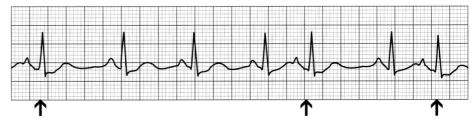

Atrial Tachycardia

A run of six or more consecutive premature atrial complexes. Atrial tachycardia results from an ectopic focus in the atria which takes over from the SA node.

May be seen with:
> Digitalis toxicity (p. 92)
> Excess catecholamines

EKG Findings

> -Atrial rate of 160-240 beats/minute.
> -First beat of rhythm is early.
> -Ectopic P waves can differ in appearance from sinus P waves.
> -Regular, constant P-R interval.
> -Normal QRS.

**Atrial tachycardia
(rate 180)**

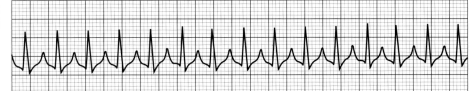

Paroxysmal Atrial Tachycardia (PAT)

PAT is atrial tachycardia with a sudden onset and an abrupt ending. "PAT with block" occurs either if the atrial rate is fast enough or if there is simultaneous AV block.

May be seen with:
> Digitalis toxicity (p. 92)
> Hypoxia
> Excessive caffeine
> Myocardial Infarction (p. 124)
> Cardiomyopathy
> Hyperthyroidism
> Hypertension
> Physical/psychological stress
> Hypokalemia (p. 94)
> Marijuana
> Congenital heart disease
> WPW syndrome (p. 112)
> Cor pulmonale (p. 109)
> Chronic Lung disease

Paroxysmal Atrial Tachycardia (cont.)

EKG Findings

-Atrial rate of 160-240 beats/minute.
-First beat of rhythm is early.
-Usually preceded by frequent premature atrial contractions.
-Ectopic P waves have abnormal configuration.
-Regular, constant P-R interval.
-Normal QRS complex.

Normal sinus rhythm with paroxysmal atrial tachycardia

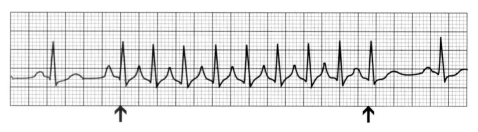

Multifocal Atrial Tachycardia (MAT)

This is sometimes referred to as Chaotic Atrial Tachycardia. It consists of a run of six or more multifocal PACs from different atrial foci. For this diagnosis to be made, three or more different configurations of P' (prime) waves must be seen.

May be seen with:
Chronic obstructive pulmonary disease
Chronic cor pulmonale (p. 109)

EKG Findings

-Early ectopic P waves.
-Irregular P-P interval.
-Irregular P-R interval.
-Non-conducted ectopic P waves may occur.
-Rate 100-200 beats/ minute.
-Normal QRS.

Multifocal atrial tachycardia

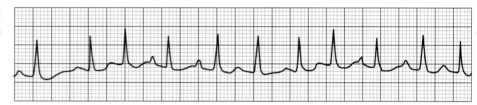

Atrial Flutter

Atrial flutter is caused by repetitive firing of atrial impulses at a rate greater than 220 beats/minute. Due to the atrial impulses occurring so rapidly, the resulting waves are called flutter waves, or F waves. The AV conduction rate is also changed, as the ventricles may only contract with every second, third or fourth beat. This results in 2:1, 3:1, or 4:1 AV conduction.

Type I Atrial Flutter (classic)—atrial rate varies between 220-350 beats/minute.

Type II Atrial Flutter—atrial rate varies between 340-430 beats/minute.

This is thought to represent an intermediate between atrial flutter and atrial fibrillation.

May be seen with:

Persons over 40 with ischemic heart disease

Pulmonary embolism (p. 105)

Thyrotoxicosis

Mitral/tricuspid valve disease

Hyperthyroidism

Atrial enlargement (p. 54)

Atrial septal defects

Chronic lung disease

Cor pulmonale (p. 109)

Digitalis toxicity (p. 92)

Pericarditis (p. 102)

Beri-beri

Atrial Flutter (cont.)

EKG Findings:
-Atrial rate greater than 220 beats/minute.
-F waves replace P waves.
-Sawtooth or picket fence pattern in leads II, III, aVF.
  -F wave is negative component of sawtooth pattern.
-Positive peaks in V1.
-P-R interval not measurable.

Atrial flutter (ventricular rate 75) 4:1 AV conduction

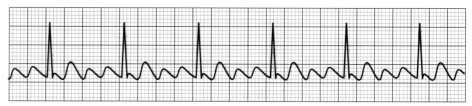

Atrial Fibrillation

Atrial fibrillation occurs when multiple ectopic foci in the atria fire repetitively at rates greater than 400 beats/minute. Due to the rapidity of these impulses, the resulting atrial contractions are weak and incomplete, and no P waves are produced. The resulting waves are called fibrillatory waves, or F waves. Fibrillatory waves may be classified as coarse or fine. The ventricular response is irregular because most of the atrial impulses fall upon a refractory AV node. This is the most common atrial tachyarrhythmia in adults. Atrial fibrillation also demonstrates Ashman's phenomenon (p. 202).

May be seen with:
>> Mitral valve disease
>> Thyrotoxicosis
>> Ischemic heart disease
>> Cardiomyopathy
>> Congestive heart failure
>> Hypertension
>> Rheumatic heart disease
>> Chronic Obstructive Pulmonary Disease

Atrial Fibrillation (cont.)

EKG Findings
-*Irregularly irregular rhythm.*
-*Atrial rate greater than 400 beats/minute.*
-*Multifocal f waves replace P waves with undulating baseline.*
-*F waves best seen in V1—this lead is closest to fibrillating atria.*
-*Irregular ventricular response.*
-*No measurable P-R interval.*
-*Wide QRS often seen secondary to aberrancy.*

Atrial fibrillation

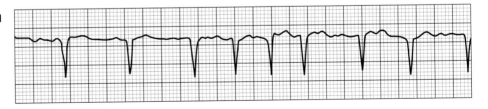

Wandering Atrial Pacemaker

Atrial dysrhythmia in which the site of impulse generation within the atria changes from beat to beat. For example, the pacemaker site may alternate between the SA and AV node; however, impulses may be generated from anywhere in atria. The rate is dependent upon pacemaker sites. When the rate exceeds 100 beats/minute, it is classified as multifocal atrial tachycardia (p. 160).

May be seen with:
> Lung disease
> Cor pulmonale (p. 109)
> Diabetes mellitus
> Digitalis toxicity (p. 92)

EKG Findings
> *-P waves vary according to pacemaker site and may be upright or inverted.*
> *-Changing P-R and R-R intervals.*
> *-Irregular rhythm.*

Wandering atrial pacemaker

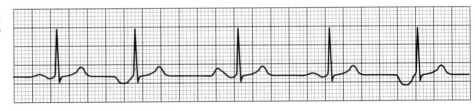

Note differences in the P waves

Premature Junctional Complexes (PJC)

PJCs are premature ectopic impulses originating from an area around the AV node or from the AV node itself. The impulses are then transmitted anterograde to the ventricles and retrograde to the atria. PJCs may be preceded by an inverted P wave, followed by an inverted P wave, or have no P wave at all. The resultant P wave inversion is due to retrograde atrial depolarization.

May be seen with:

> Digitalis toxicity (p. 92)
> Myocardial ischemia (p. 120)
> Myocardial Infarction (p. 124)
> Adrenergic tone (e.g., Excessive caffeine/amphetamine intake)

EKG Findings

> -Ectopic beat is premature.
> -Inverted P waves preceding or following QRS.
> -If P wave follows QRS complex, T wave may be distorted.
> -Inverted, ectopic P wave falls either before, after, or within QRS complex.
>   (if no P wave is present, this indicates that either no atrial depolarization occurred or that the P
>   wave is hidden in the QRS complex).
> -If P-R interval is present, will be < 0.12 sec.
> -Usually normal narrow QRS.
> -May take the form of AV dissociation (escape rhythm).

**Normal sinus rhythm
with premature
junctional contractions**

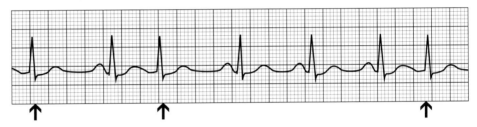

Junctional Escape Beat

Usually arises from the AV node. These impulses are generated if the SA node does not fire and a pause ensues. An escape beat from the AV node prevents asystole from occurring. The impulses are transmitted anterograde to the ventricles and retrograde to the atria. The escape beats may be isolated with a resumption of SA node firing, or may occur in pairs or runs.

EKG Findings

-Ectopic beat occurs late in cycle (as opposed to PJC which occurs early).
-Preceded by either inverted P wave, no P wave, or sinus P wave with short P-R interval (if no P wave present, indicates either no atrial depolarization or P wave in the QRS complex).
-P waves usually inverted in I, II, III, and upright in aVR.
-Normal QRS duration.

Junctional escape beat

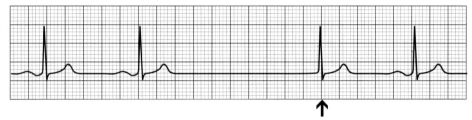

Junctional Escape Rhythm

This is a run of 6 or more consecutive junctional escape beats with a rate varying between 40-60 beats/minute. This is also called a junctional rhythm. This may occur when the SA node fails to fire or if there is a blockage in the conduction system or when there is enhanced AV Nodal (junctional) automaticity.

EKG Findings

-First beat of escape rhythm is late.

-Inverted ectopic P wave in I, II, III, and upright in aVR.

-P wave may precede or follow QRS (if no P wave present, indicates either no atrial depolarization or P wave in QRS complex) or sinus P wave may precede QRS with a shortened P-R interval—indicates lack of conduction of P wave.

-Normal QRS duration.

-Rate 40-60 beats/minute.

Junctional escape rhythm (rate 50)

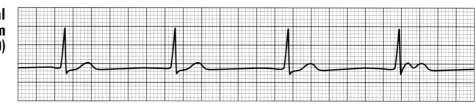

Accelerated Junctional Rhythm
Rate between 60-100 beats/minute (p. 174).

Junctional Tachycardia
Rate between 100-160 beats/minute (p. 175).

Accelerated Junctional Tachycardia
Rate greater than 160 beats/minute (p. 175).

Accelerated junctional rhythm

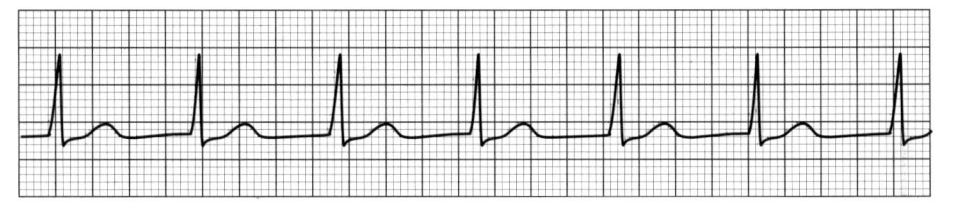

**Junctional
tachycardia**

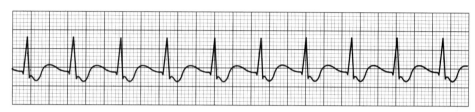

**Accelerated
junctional
tachycardia**

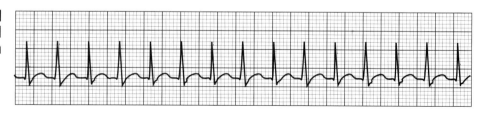

Paroxysmal Junctional Tachycardia

This has an abrupt onset and termination. The rate varies between 140-200 beats/minute.
May be seen with:

> Coronary artery disease
> Rheumatic heart disease
> Hypertension
> Digitalis toxicity (p. 92)

EKG Findings

> -*Abrupt onset and termination.*
> -*Rate 140-200 beats/minute.*
> -*Normal QRS.*

Paroxysmal junctional tachycardia (rate 180)

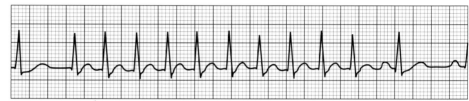

Atrioventricular Nodal Reentry Tachycardia

This is the most common cause of paroxysmal supraventricular tachycardia. AV nodal reentry involves two separate pathways; a slow pathway with a short refractory period, and a fast pathway which has a long refractory period. These are named alpha and beta pathways, respectively. The long refractory period of the beta pathway mimics a unidirectional block. An impulse travels anterograde down the slow pathway; by the time it makes its way down this pathway, the fast pathway has had time to repolarize, thus allowing for retrograde transmission of the impulse. This is known as reentry, and may result in a circus-type rhythm.

> #### EKG Findings
> -Narrow QRS duration.
> -Aberrancy uncommon.
> -P' wave may be buried in QRS complex.
> -May see r' or R' in V1.
> -Negative P' wave in leads II, III, aVF.
> -Often have a long initiating P'-R interval.

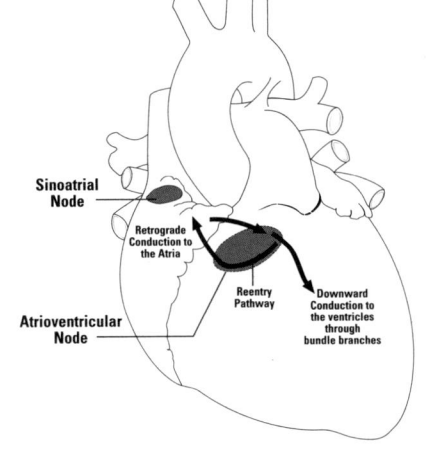

**AV nodal
reentry
tachycardia**

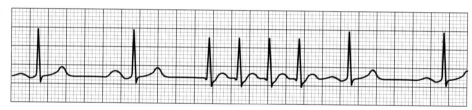

Premature Ventricular Complexes (PVC)

PVCs are early ectopic beats which emanate from the ventricles and depolarize the myocardium. These impulses spread through the ventricles with some delay since conduction through the myocardial muscle is slower than that through the conduction pathways. The atrial cycle may continue independently of the PVCs.

EKG Findings

-P wave usually lost—exception: if there is retrograde conduction to atria, may have inverted P wave following QRS.
-Widened and bizarre QRS, at least 0.12 seconds duration.
-T waves opposite in direction to QRS complexes.
-Obscured S-T segments.
-No measurable P-R interval.

EKG Appearances of PVCs:

Uniform (Unifocal)—all PVCs originate from same focus and have identical QRS complexes.
Multiform (Multifocal)—PVCs originate from different foci and have QRS complexes that differ in appearance.

**Normal sinus rhythm
with
uniform PVCs**

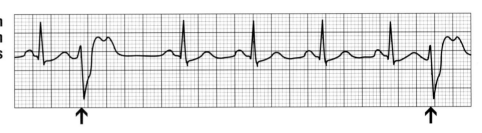

**Normal sinus rhythm
with
multiform PVCs**

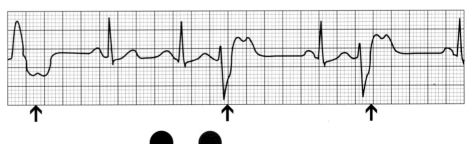

Premature Ventricular Complexes (cont.)

    Interpolated PVC: located between 2 normal sinus beats without a compensatory pause.

    R on T phenomenon: PVC that falls on T wave of previous beat. Makes heart vulnerable to repetitive firing from
    that focus leading to dangerous arrhythmias. The implacations of R on T phenomenon are controversial.

    Couplets: two identical PVCs which occur in pairs.

**Normal sinus rhythm
with
uniform PVCs**

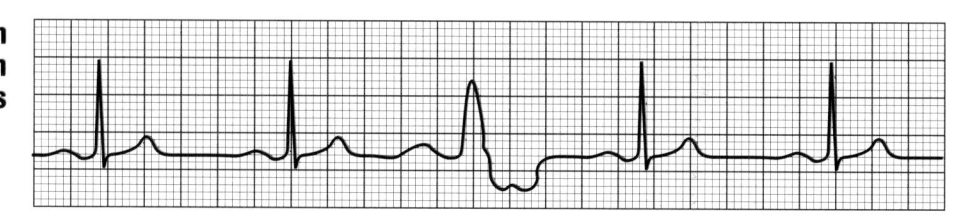

**Normal sinus rhythm
with
uniform PVCs**

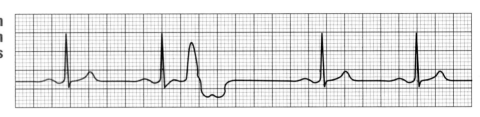

**Normal sinus rhythm
with
PVC couplet**

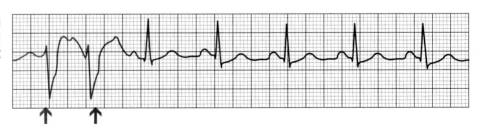

Premature Ventricular Complexes (cont.)

    Bigeminy: a repeating pattern of one normal beat followed by one uniform PVC.

    Trigeminy: as in bigeminy, with PVC occurring after two normal beats.

    Ventricular Tachycardia: by definition, 3 or more PVCs in a row (also called a salvo).

    Note: Some authors define bigeminy as every sinus beat being followed by a PVC, and trigeminy as each
    sinus beat being followed by two PVCs (*Practical Electrocardiography*, Marriot, Henry J.L., 8th ed., 1988, p.142)

**Ventricular
bigeminy**

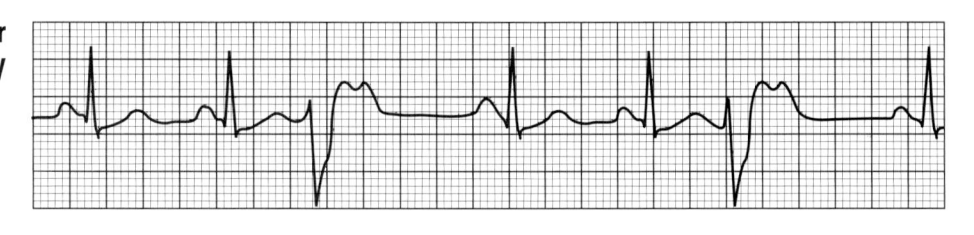

**Ventricular
trigeminy**

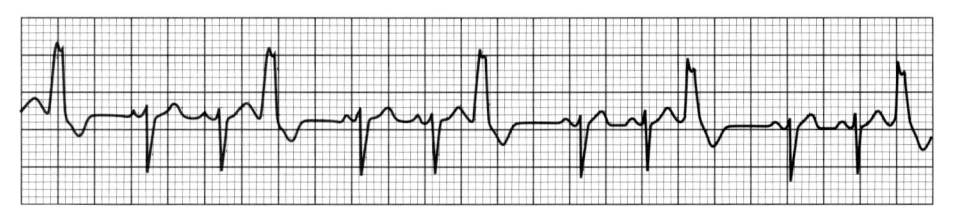

Pauses:

Full Compensatory Pause—interval between QRS preceding and following PVC is 2 times that of a normal cycle.

Partial Compensatory Pause—interval between QRS preceding and following PVC is less than 2 times that of a normal cycle.

Full compensatory pause

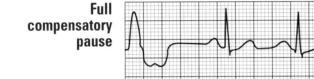

2x normal cycle

Partial compensatory pause

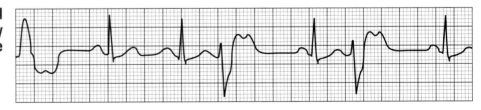

Premature Ventricular Complexes (cont.)
   Lown's Grading System of Ventricular Ectopy: This grading system is used for predicting the risk of death following myocardial infarction. The risk of death increases as the numerical grade increases.

GRADE	GRADING OF VENTRICULAR PREMATURE BEATS
0	No ventricular premature beats
1	Occasional, isolated (30/hour)
1A	less than 1/min.
1B	more than 1/min.
2	30 or more/hour
3	Multiform
4A	Two consecutive
4B	3 or more consecutive
5	R-on-T

(Ref. Lown, B., and Graboys, T.B.: *Management of Patients with Malignant Ventricular Arrhythmias.* Am. J. Cardiol. 1977: 39, 910.)

   Note: Modifications of this grading scheme have been made, and there is debate about the relative dangers of the different grades. However, many articles make reference to this original scheme.

Premature Ventricular Complexes (cont.)

PVCs may be seen with:
Idiopathic
Emotional stress
Hypokalemia (p. 94)
Hypocalcemia (p. 98)
Digitalis toxicity (p. 92)
Ingestion of stimulants—i.e., caffeine, tobacco, alcohol
Ingestion of medications—i.e., epinephrine, isoproterenol, theophylline
Ischemia

Ventricular Tachycardia

This consists of three or more PVCs in a row. Also called a salvo. The depolarizing focus occurs in one ventricle and spreads to the adjacent ventricle following a short delay; this results in wide, bizarre QRS complexes. Firing of SA node may continue independently of ventricular depolarization; this is called AV dissociation (p. 202). The most reliable sign of ventricular tachycardia is the <u>capture beat</u>, also called the <u>Dressler beat</u>. This occurs when an impulse originating from the SA node is conducted through the AV node to the ventricles and the resulting normal QRS complex is seen within a run of ventricular tachycardia. A less reliable sign often seen is a <u>fusion beat</u>. This is a normal sinus impulse which is produced simultaneously with the ectopic ventricular impulse. Resulting QRS complex appears as an intermediate between a normally produced QRS and a QRS of ventricular origin.

May be seen with:

Myocardial infarction	Ischemic heart disease
Mitral valve prolapse	Cardiomyopathies
Digitalis toxicity (p. 92)	Idiopathic

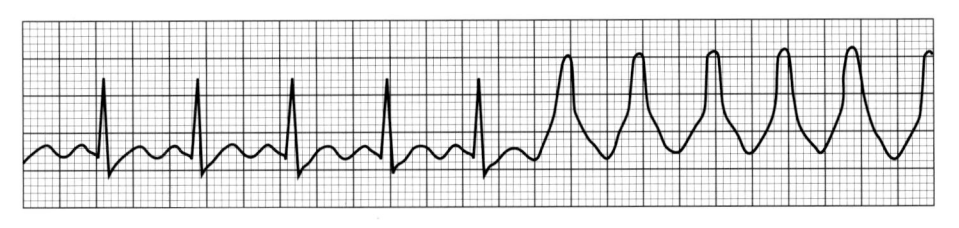

Sinus Tachycardia changing to Ventricular tachycardia

Ventricular Tachycardia (cont.)

EKG Findings

-First beat of rhythm is early.
-Rate between 100-220 beats/minute.
-Greater than 3 PVCs in a row.
-No ectopic P waves (however, these may be seen with AV dissociation).
-No measurable P-R interval.
-Wide, bizarre QRS complexes (>0.12 sec).
-May see following QRS complexes:
   lead V1- RR' (R'>R), qR, Rs
   lead V6- qR, QS
-Left axis deviation in > 75% of patients.
-Slightly irregular rate.

Ventricular Flutter

One or more ventricular foci firing rapidly and repetitively with a fairly regular rate and rhythm. Rate varies between 150-250 beats/minute. Considered an intermediary between ventricular tachycardia and ventricular fibrillation

Ventricular Fibrillation

Consists of multiple ventricular foci firing rapidly and repetitively causing disorganized ventricular contractions. Ventricular rate can vary between 150-500 beats/minute. No P waves or QRS complexes can be discerned.

May be seen with:

Sudden Cardiac Death
Untreated ventricular tachycardia
R on T phenomenon
Congenital heart disease
Ischemic heart disease
Drug effects

Existing heart disease
Hypothermia (p. 104)
Cardiomyopathy
Electri shock
Metabolic abnormalities

EKG Findings

-No identifiable P waves, T waves, or QRS complexes.
-Rate usually indeterminable-usually 150-500 beats/minute.
-Irregular rhythm.
-May be coarse or fine ventricular fibrillation.

Ventricular fibrillation

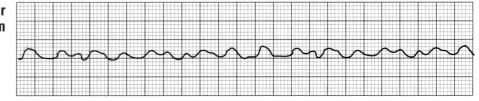

Torsade de Pointes (tor-sahd'-de-pwahnt)

This is a special form of polymorphous ventricular tachycardia. The name means twisting around the point. It can be regarded as a combination of ventricular tachycardia and ventricular fibrillation. The exact etiology and mechanism are unknown. It is believed to be a form of reentry. The QRS polarity alternates between positive and negative beats around an isoelectric baseline. Usual antiarrhythmic drugs are contraindicated as they aggravate the arrhythmia.

May be seen with:

> Certain medications—quinidine, procainamide, disopyramide, phenothiazines
> Electrolyte disturbances, especially low magnesium
> Insecticide poisoning
> Congenital Q-T prolongation
> AV block (p. 210)
> Subarachnoid hemorrhage (p. 116)
> Bradycardia

EKG Findings

> -*Wide, bizarre QRS complexes.*
> -*Alternating positive and negative polarity of beats.*

Torsade de Pointes

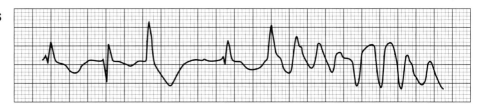

Idioventricular Rhythm

This is also called a ventricular escape rhythm. It consists of six or more consecutive ventricular escape beats (p. 197) at rate of less than 40 beats/minute. This occurs when the SA node fails to fire or when there is a blockage of the conduction system.

EKG Findings

-First beat of rhythm is late.
-No ectopic P waves.
-Wide, bizarre QRS.
-Rate less than 40 beats/minute.

Idioventricular rhythm (rate 35)

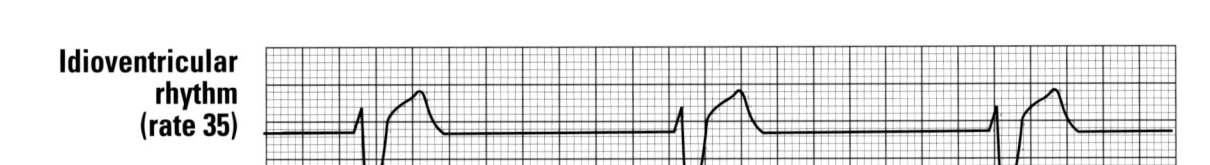

Ventricular Escape Beat

If a long pause occurs, a ventricular focus will sometimes fire spontaneously to reinstate a rhythm.

Ventricular escape

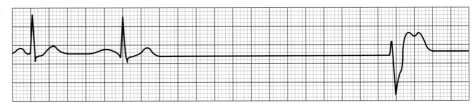

Accelerated Idioventricular Rhythm (AIVR)

This rhythm has a rate usually between 40-100 beats/minute. Most episodes last only seconds to minutes. May be seen with:

> Digitalis intoxication (p. 92)
> Myocardial infarction (p. 124)
> Sinus bradycardia (p. 146)
> Reperfusion rhythms

EKG Findings

-Ventricular rate slower than ventricular tachycardia.

-Wide, bizarre QRS complexes.

-Short duration: seconds to minutes.

-No ectopic P waves.

-T wave usually opposite in direction of QRS.

**Accelerated
idioventricular
rhythm**

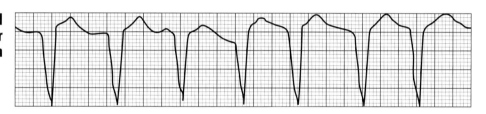

Parasystole

An ectopic pacemaker, most commonly ventricular, which fires impulses at a regular rate concurrently and usually slower than dominant pacemaker rhythm. The ectopic focus is protected by either entrance or exit block. A fusion beat (see p. 185) may result if the parasystolic impulse is fired at the same time as the sinus node impulse. The parasystolic focus is inextinguishable. Parasystolic impulses will not be seen if they encounter a refractory conduction pathway.

May be seen with:

> Elderly patients
> Idiopathic
> Myocardial infarction (p. 124)

EKG Findings

> *-Irregular rhythm as result of parasystolic beats.*
> *-Abnormal P wave may result depending on location of parasystolic focus.*
> *-QRS complex may vary depending on location of parasystolic focus.*
> *-Varying distance between the ventricular beats and the preceding normal beats (variable coupling).*

Parasystole

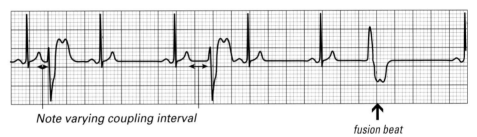

Note varying coupling interval

fusion beat

Atrioventricular Dissociation

In AV dissociation the atria and ventricles are controlled by different pacemakers and beat independently of each other. The atria are depolarized by firing of an atrial focus and the ventricles are depolarized by firing of an ectopic focus either in the AV node or in the ventricle. This is considered to be a double rhythm. AV dissociation is usually caused by one or more of the following mechanisms: 1) slowing of sinoatrial node, i.e., bradycardia; 2) blockade of sinus impulses in sinoatrial node or in atrioventricular node; 3) acceleration of ectopic pacemaker site, i.e., accelerated idioventricular rhythm, junctional tachycardia, ventricular tachycardia 4) any rhythm producing a pause, i.e., extrasystoles, ending of tachycardia. Complete heart block is one type of AV dissociation (see p. 81).

May be seen with:

> Atrioventricular block (p. 210)
> Ventricular tachycardia (p. 188)
> Complete heart block (p. 84)
> Sinus arrest (p. 152)
> Junctional tachycardia (p. 176)
> Sinus bradycardia
> Digitalis toxicity (p. 92)
> Sinoatrial block (p. 150)
> Any combination of above conditions

Atrioventricular Dissociation (cont.)

EKG Findings

-Atria and ventricles beat regularly, but independently of each other.

-Regular P-P intervals.

-Regular R-R intervals.

-No relationship between P-P and R-R intervals.

-No relationship between P waves and QRS complexes.

AV dissociation

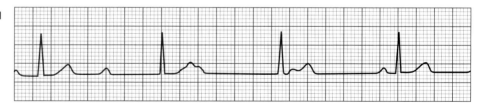

Aberrancy

Aberrancy, or aberration, is recognized by a temporary variation in the normal QRS configuration. This occurs when a sinus or supraventricular impulse stimulates the ventricles in an abnormal way. This is usually the result of a transmitted impulse encountering a refractory bundle branch; the impulse is then abnormally transmitted from one ventricle to the other, most commonly through the myocardium. Due to this delayed transmission, a wide, bizarre QRS in seen. The most common causes of aberration occur when a premature atrial complex or a junctional premature complex occurs too close to the preceding beat, thus encountering a bundle branch which is still in a partially refractory state. This may also be seen in atrial fibrillation. One etiology of aberrancy is **Ashman's phenomenon**. This is defined as aberrant conduction caused by changing R-R intervals. A longer R-R interval will result in a longer bundle branch refractory period. If this is followed by a shorter R-R interval, the resulting impulse may encounter a bundle branch which is still refractory; this leads to aberrant conduction.

Aberrancy (cont.)

EKG Findings
-Premature atrial complex with aberrancy.
  -early ectopic P wave preceding wide, bizarre QRS complex.
-OR premature junctional complex with aberrancy.
  -inverted, early, ectopic P wave preceding or immediately following wide, bizarre QRS complex.
-OR atrial fibrillation with aberrancy.
  -long R-R cycle followed by short R-R cycle followed by wide, bizarre QRS complex.

PAC with aberrancy

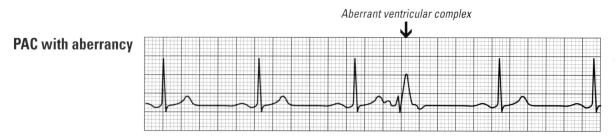

Aberrant ventricular complex

Differentiating the wide QRS tachycardias

Wide QRS complexes may result from impulses originating from either ventricular or supraventricular foci. Ventricular tachycardia is the most common of wide QRS tachycardias. However, this must be differentiated from wide QRS tachycardia of supraventricular origin, as the treatments of these two entities differs. Wide QRS complexes of supraventricular origin may be seen in the following situations:

1) with pre-existing right or left bundle branch block. The supraventricular impulse encounters a refractory bundle branch due to the block and this results in delayed intraventricular conduction time (p. 70).

2) impulse conduction into ventricles across one or more anomalous pathways (i.e., Wolff-Parkinson-White Syndrome [p. 112]).

3) drug-induced defective intraventricular conduction. Wide QRS complexes of ventricular origin result in abnormal impulse propagation and conduction (see ventricular tachycardia p. 188).

Note: When discussing QRS complexes, capital letters refer to waves which are proportionally larger than those assigned small cased letters.

Differentiating the wide QRS tachycardias (cont.)

EKG Findings which may aid in differentiating wide complex tachycardias:

<u>Suggestive of Ventricular origin</u>:
-rate less than 140 beats/min.
-QRS duration greater than 0.14 sec.
-left axis deviation (greater than -30°)
-lead V1: R > R' **OR** broad R wave
        OR Rsr' **OR** qR **OR** QR **OR** RS
-lead V6: small q, large R or QS
-AV dissociation (see pages 199-200)
-fusion beats (p. 209)

<u>Suggestive of Supraventricular origin</u>:
-rate greater than 170 beats/min.
-QRS duration less than 0.12 sec. with RBBB
-QRS duration less than 0.14 sec. with LBBB
-lead V1: RSR' OR rSR' -this can also be seen with
    ventricular origin, but is usually supraventricular)
-lead V6: qRs

Ventricular Fusion

Fusion Beats

Fusion beats occur when impulses from two different foci simultaneously activate the ventricles. Most commonly these are comprised of an SA node impulse and a premature ventricular complex, although the beats may originate anywhere in the heart. The resulting complex seen on electrocardiogram is usually a hybrid of the two beats. Fusion beats are reliable indicators that the rhythm is at least partly ventricular in origin.

EKG Findings
-Bizarre, wide QRS complex.
-T wave usually bizarre in appearance.
-Contains features which are intermediates of the two impulses comprising the fused beat.

Fusion beat

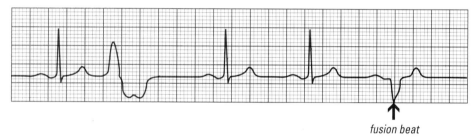

fusion beat

Atrio-Ventricular Heart Block

First-Degree Heart Block
Most common conduction disturbance. It is caused by an increase delay at the level of the AV node. Therefore, it takes longer for each atrial impulse to reach the myocardium. This is manifested by a prolonged P-R interval.

May be seen with:

Acute myocarditis
Hyperkalemia (p. 96)
Mild digitalis toxicity (p. 92)
Acute myocardial infarction (p. 124)
Most common and earliest finding in
acute conduction system disease,
e.g., Lev's disease

Hypothyroid
Collagen vascular disease
Cardiomyopathies
Chronic aortic regurgitation

EKG Findings
-Fixed, prolonged P-R interval > 0.20 in adults and > 0.18 in children.
-Constant P-R interval.
-Regular rhythm.
-Normal P waves.
-Normal QRS complexes.

First-degree AV block

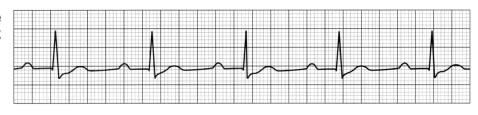

Second-Degree Heart Block

Ventricles do not respond to all atrial stimuli and not all P waves are followed by QRS complexes. Subdivided into Mobitz type I (Wenckebach) and Mobitz type II.

Mobitz type I (Wenckebach)

Usually indicates an atrioventricular intranodal block. Characterized by progressively increasing P-R intervals until P wave is not followed by QRS complex. This is due to lengthening of the refractory period until P wave impulse is blocked from depolarizing the ventricles. The Wenckebach phenomenon or Wenckebach period is defined as the progressive lengthening of the P-R interval, followed by a P wave without a QRS. Wenckebach is generally a benign rhythm.

May be seen with:

Ischemic heart disease	Intense vagal stimulation
Rheumatic fever	Inferior wall MI (p. 138)
Digitalis toxicity (p. 92)	Electrolyte imbalance (transient)
Cardiomyopathies	Primary conduction system disease
Beta blockers	Calcium channel blockers

EKG Findings

-Progressive lengthening of P-R interval until QRS-T complex is dropped.
-Shortening of R-R interval.
-Normal P waves.
-Normal QRS complexes.

Second-degree AV block Type I (Wenckebach)

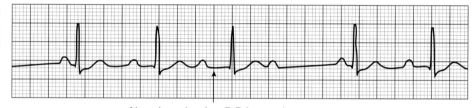

Note lengthening P-R interval

Second-Degree Heart Block (cont.)

Mobitz type II
Usually indicates atrioventricular infranodal block. Less common than Mobitz type I AV block. Characterized by blocked P wave without preceding Wenckebach period. Block in conduction system is located distal to AV node; therefore, QRS may be prolonged and widened.

May be seen with:

Anterior/anteroseptal myocardial infarction or ischemia (p. 134)

EKG Findings
-*Constant P-R interval in conducted beats.*
-*Widened QRS complexes due to intraventricular conduction delay.*
-*Occasional dropped QRS-T complex.*
-*Constant R-R intervals in conducted beats.*
-*P-P interval containing non-conducted P wave equal to two normal P-P intervals.*

Second-degree AV block Type II

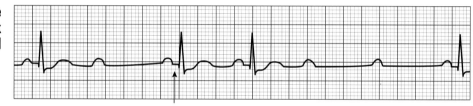

Note that the P-R interval doesn't change

Third-Degree Heart Block (Complete Heart Block)

Due to a complete block in the area of the atrioventricular junction or along the ventricular conduction pathways, no atrial impulses are conducted to the ventricles. Therefore, a secondary pacemaker takes over the pacing of the ventricles. This secondary pacemaker may be located anywhere distal to the area of the blockage (see junctional escape beat p. 170, ventricular escape beat p. 195). Ventricular rhythm is usually a bradycardia. No retrograde impulses can reach the atria due to the block.

May be seen with:

Acute anterior MI (p. 134)	Any cause of 1st- or 2nd-degree heart block
Myocardial ischemia (p. 120)	Acute inferior walll MI (p. 138)
Rheumatic fever	Electrolyte imbalances
Congenital	Digitalis toxicity (p. 92)
Cardiomyopathy	Diphtheria

Lev's disease (fibrosis and calcification spreading from valves or septum to the conductive tissue-produces bilateral bundle branch block)

Lenegre's disease (fibrosis of conductive tissue-produces bilateral bundle branch block)

Third-Degree Heart Block (cont.)

EKG Findings

-Independent atrial and ventricular pacing.
-P-P intervals usually regular.
-R-R intervals usually regular.
-No relationship between P-P and R-R intervals.
-No relationship between P waves and QRS complexes.
-Ventricular rate usually <45 beats/minute.
-Escape rhythm QRS complex may be either narrow or wide.

Third-degree block

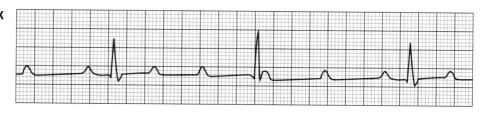

References

- Conover, Mary B. *Understanding Electrocardiography, Arrhythmias and the 12-lead ECG.* 7th ed. C. V. Mosby Company, 1996

- Johnson, Richard and Swartz, Mark. *A Simplified Approach to Electrocardiography.* W. B. Saunders Company, 1986.

- Marriott, Henry J. *Pearls and Pitfalls in Electrocardiography: Pithy, Practical Pointers.* 2nd Edition. John Wiley and Sons, 1998.

- Phibbs, Brandon P. *Advanced ECG: Boards and Beyond: What You Really Need to Know About Electrocardiography.* Little Brown and Company, 1996.

- Thaler, Malcolm S. *The Only EKG Book You'll Ever Need.* 3rd Edition. Lippincott, Williams and Wilkins Publishers, 1999.

- Wagner, Galen S. and Marriott, Henry J. *Practical Electrocardiography.* 9th Edition. Williams and Wilkins, 1994.

Index

Index